HISTORY OF MEDICINE IN BROWN COUNTY, WISCONSIN 1816-2000

A TRANSITION

INDEPENDENT MEDICAL PRACTITIONER TO MULTISPECIALTY CLINIC PROVIDER

B.L. Richardson MD

Illustrations by William F. Schneider MD

Publisher's Cataloging-in-Publication
(Provided by Quality Books, Inc.)

Richardson, B. L.
History of medicine in Brown County, Wisconsin 1816-2000 : a transition : independent medical practitioner to multispecialty clinic provider / B.L. Richardson ; illustrations by William F. Schneider. -- 1st ed.
p. cm.
Includes bibliographical references and index.
LCCN: 2002112079
ISBN: 0972406409

1. Medicine--Wisconsin--Brown County--History.
2. Physicians--Wisconsin--Brown County--Biography.
3. Brown County (Wis.)--Biography. I. Title.

R358.B76R53 2002 610'.9'77561
QBI02-200672

Dedicated to the Brown County Medical Society whose members, past and present, have actively participated in the medical, political, and economic issues of the day. Special recognition should be reserved for those who gave of their unique talents and time to lead the Wisconsin Medical Society.

TABLE OF CONTENTS

Preface

My interest in the history of medicine in Brown County began in the doctors' lounge of the hospital. The doctors' lounge was a convenient setting for informal discussion of current cases and the economics of medical practice. It also was a classroom for history. I learned much about the more prominent doctors who had at one time or another practiced in the area. The more experienced physicians would enjoy telling stories of the "old days." It was tantamount to an oral history that was confined to the fraternity of practicing physicians. An the end of a session, of usually scandalous tales, the comment was often made that someone ought to document the history because details would soon be lost.

Two surgeons who had practiced early in the twentieth century were most often the subject of the impromptu history lessons. But as I was to discover, there is much more to the history of medicine in Brown County than the verbal legends of Drs. Minhan and Bellin. The only previous history published was a brief article in the 1929 Wisconsin State Medical Journal by Dr. Thomas Oliver. Dr. Oliver identified many of the early doctors and made pertinent comments on the hospitals.

Published articles and books by others in Wisconsin do not reflect the details of Brown County medicine, despite the fact that the first Wisconsin physicians practiced in this area. Most histories concentrate on Southern Wisconsin and ignore Brown County physicians other than Dr. William Beaumont.

Research revealed a wealth of sources harboring hidden facts. Those sources were found with the invaluable assistance of many individuals. Mary Jane Herber of the Brown County Historical Library, in addition to her extensive knowledge of Brown County history, was especially helpful in indicating where to locate material. Sister Ann Bailey, Archivist of the Third Order of St. Francis, was most encouraging during a visit to the Mother House in Springfield, Illinois. Liliane Theriault, of the Misericorde Order, cordially responded to my requests for information concerning St. Mary's Hospital. Deborah Anderson, of the UWGB Library, Mike Duplaise, from St. Mary's Hospital, Larry Hohol of Bellin Hospital, and Micaela Sullivan-Fowler of the University of Wisconsin Middelton Medical Library each graciously gave of their time and expertise. I am also indebted to Betsy Foley for her knowledgeable advice and encouragement and to my daughter, Karen Admussen, for reviewing the manuscript. The insight and personal involvement of associates who consented to interviews was much appreciated.

Dr. William Schneider's drawings are especially valued as they reflect his accomplished artistic ability and a genuine interest in history. The illustrations are based upon exhibits from the Fort Howard Museum and Heritage Hill Collections located in Green Bay, Wisconsin.

Julie Wilhm is acknowledged for excellent work and artistic design of the book jacket.

The advise and counsel of Dawn Jeffers from Raven Tree Press was invaluable in publishing and without the financial support of the Brown County Medical Society this whole project may have been buried in the unpublished papers that can be found among the effects of many physicians.

My sincere apologies to those physicians who practiced or who are currently practicing in Brown County who are not identified in this history. Over four hundred doctors are now in Brown County and it was impossible to document the names and achievements of all.

As I became more familiar with the men and women who had practiced medicine in Brown County, through newspaper articles, medical journal writings, interviews, and autobiographical manuscripts, a greater appreciation of the intellect, courage, compassion and dedication of these physicians emerged. I could more fully appreciate that the profound changes in medical knowledge, technology, and clinical practice structure have not altered the basic underlying motivation of the Brown County physician.

Benson Lee Richardson MD

Time Line

Fort Howard Hospital	1816
St. Vincent Hospital	1888
St. Mary's Mothers' and Infants' Home	1900
St. Mary's Hospital	1903
Deaconess Sanitarium (Bellin Hospital)	1908
Green Bay Clinic	1929
St. Vincent Ten Story Addition	1957
Goelz Clinic (Deckner)	1958
St. Mary's Moves to West Side	1960
West Side Clinic	1960
Beaumont Clinic	1962
Lynn Clinic (Webster)	1962
Dousman Clinic	1970
Bellin Adds Van Buren Building	1977
New West Side St. Mary's Hospital	1981
Bay Care	1994
Bellin Medical Group	1994
Aurora Medical Group	1994
Prevea Clinic	1994
Bay Care Aurora Hospital (Proposed)	1999

Presidents of Wisconsin State Medical Society

Dr. Cooper Ayres 1856-57

Dr. Benjamin Brett 1893-94

Dr. Ralph Carter 1935-36

Dr. P. R. Minahan 1945-46

Dr. A. J. McCarey 1954-55

Dr. John Dettmann 1974-75

Dr. Roger VON Heimburg 1990-91

Illustrations and Photographs

Hospitals

Physicians

Illustrations

HISTORY OF MEDICINE IN BROWN COUNTY, WISCONSIN 1816-2000

Chapter 1

Military Doctors

The first practitioners of the healing arts, in what is now known as Brown County, Wisconsin, were the American Indian medicine men. The American Indian believed that life was in balance or in disharmony. Illness was an imbalance or disharmony that may be directly related to spiritual causes. Life was a sacred circle. There was no beginning or end. Everything was related to nature and the world of spirits. Indian healers looked beyond the symptoms to discover the root of illness. Disease could be due to natural, human, or supernatural origins. Equilibrium was lost due to grief, sadness, or personal wrongdoing. Healing would bring the person back to balance. Most illness was related to hunger, exposure, fevers, or wounds. Severe contagious diseases were introduced by the white settlers. The medicine men used herbs in concert with religious ceremony in their practice. [1] This was holistic medicine.

Each tribe had its own collection of herbal medicines. Some used blood root leaves to relieve indigestion. The root of the yellow water lily was used to make a poultice for cuts and bruises. The inner bark of the slippery elm could draw pus from a wound and the root of the trillium could treat swollen eyelids. Wild prairie parsley was used for respiratory illness. Other plants that are mentioned include echinacea, ginseng, evening primrose, saw palmetto, and cranberry juice. Whether the Winnebago, Menominee, and Fox tribes used these herbs is not well documented but is likely. Ceremony might include dance, prayers, the beating of drums, and the wearing of a mask to ward off evil spirits. The pike fish tooth might be used to pick the skin and draw blood for introducing medication into the body. The sweat bath was used for cleansing, purification and spiritual strengthening. Women acted as midwives and sometimes bone setters. Wounds were carefully dressed and poultices applied. According to one early white settler's account, the Indian healer was more successful in treating wounds than the early surgeons. [2]

Training to be a medicine man was through apprenticeship. The secrets of healing were purposely confined to only a few and passed down through the generations. A fee for services, in some instances, was given before the administration to the sick but was returned if the patient was unimproved or treatment unsuccessful. Healing was a spiritual phenomenon aided by medicines available to the Indian from his natural environment.

Jean Nicolet in 1634 was the first white explorer to visit the mouth of the Fox

River. He was followed by Nicolas Perrot, 1665, Father Claude Allouez, 1669, and the French military. A fort was built on the west side of the Fox River in 1706 to protect French territorial and trade interests. The French were engaged in action against bands of hostile Indians for almost 30 years. There are no records of French surgeons residing at the fort during this time.

It wasn't until 1745 that the first permanent settler arrived. Augustin De Langlade made his home on the eastern shore of the Fox River opposite the French fort. The settlers aligned themselves with the friendly Indians and French against the British, who were attempting to push their domain westward and command rewards of the fur trade. The British subsequently defeated the French and Indian warriors. The treaty which followed gave Britain the Northwest Territory. This included the area later designated as Brown County. British troops took possession of the French Fort in 1761. After the English defeat in the Revolutionary War, the area was ceded to the United States. By 1810, there were about fifty settlers on either side of the Fox River. Their log cabins were located upstream from the mouth of the river all the way to Kaukauna. A Menominee Indian village was present on the east bank of the Fox River.

During the War of 1812, the British took over Fort Mackinac and control of the territory. Dr. David Mitchell, a British Army surgeon and a graduate of Edinburgh University, was assigned in 1813-1814 to the Indian Service at Lake Winnebago.[3] After Dr. Mitchell left the area, the nearest physician was at Fort Machinac 200 miles away. If someone was sick or injured, he had to survive a trip to the Fort or rely upon the skills of friends and the use of natural remedies for medical care. Many families kept a stock of roots and herbs for treatment of the common ailments.

United States Congress, following the War of 1812, authorized the army to build military posts at Green Bay, Prairie Du Chien, and Portage, Wisconsin. These posts were to protect the interests of the fur traders and the settlers. In 1816 Colonel J. Miller landed on the shores of the Fox River and decided to build a fort at the site of the original French outpost. Dr. William Henry Hening, the regimental surgeon, accompanied the troops but did not stay and most likely left with Colonel Miller. The fortification was named Fort Howard after General Benjamin Howard, a hero of the War of 1812.

Dr. William Madison arrived in 1819 after Fort Howard was constructed. He was the first American physician to be stationed in the territory. The hospital was a log structure, originally used as a stable and converted to use for the surgeon. The hospital was located outside of the fort stockade, presumably, to isolate the sick from the healthy troops. Little is known about Dr. Madison's practice. He was in the military service prior to arriving at Fort Howard. Unfortunately, he met an untimely death in 1821.

Dr. Madison had taken an Indian wife as was the practice of many of the settlers. He decided to temporarily leave his Native American wife in the area and visit his white wife and new baby who lived in Kentucky. He was accompanied on his trip by two soldiers and Ke-tau-ka, brother of his Indian wife. They had left Green Bay and had stopped for the evening near Manitowoc. Without obvious provocation, Dr. Madison was shot by Ke-tau-ka. The reasons for the shooting have varied. Ke-tau-ka may have been angry because the doctor was leaving his Indian wife or another report suggested that the act was committed because a band of Indians camped near the doctor's camp would not allow Ke-tau-ka to participate in their game of throwing an axe at a post unless he could claim he killed a white man. Allegedly, to join in the activity , he shot the doctor. Dr. Madison died May 14, 1821 before the soldiers could transport him back to the fort. The band of Indians turned Ke-tau-ka over to the soldiers and eventually he was tried, convicted, and hanged for the offense. [4]

In addition to the post surgeon, an assistant surgeon was on occasion assigned to Fort Howard. The harsh climate was thought to be responsible for a high incidence of sickness.

J. P. MacMahon and H. F. Hall, assistant surgeons, appear briefly on the report of personnel assigned to Fort Howard in 1819 and 1821 respectively. It is likely they were not present very long.

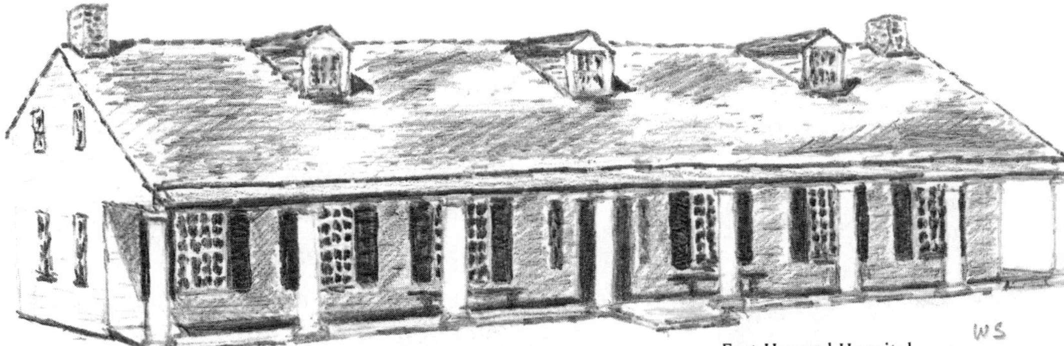

Fort Howard Hospital

In 1823 Dr. Walter Wheaton became the post surgeon. He was joined by Dr. Richard Satterlee on his first brief tour at Fort Howard. Dr. Wheaton was frequently called upon to administer to the settlers. There were about fifty families, predominantly of French background, many married to Indian women, living on the east bank of the Fox River in 1820. Settlers were treated at the hospital or sometimes in their homes. The civilians knew they could go to the fort hospital and find the surgeon. The official army inspector's report stated that "the hospital was in good order. The hospital stores and medicines abundant, of good quality, and well arranged, creditable to surgeon Wheaton and assistant Satterlee who are vigilant and skillful." It was reported that thirty-four men were ill, mostly convalescent. [5]

The fort was often the setting for the social life of the families living on the east side of the river as well as the military. Dinners, dancing, and theatrical productions helped occupy the long winter nights. On one occasion, Dr. Wheaton decided to attend a social gathering in Kaukauna. He traveled by sleigh, as it was winter. He apparently stayed a few extra days and upon returning to Fort Howard discovered one of the soldiers had been operated upon by his eighteen-year-old brother.

The account of this incident is a reflection of the primitive and often brutal nature of frontier medicine. Records indicate Lieutenant Morgan and a man named Webster were going north on Green Bay to procure fish and supplies for the Fort. They were caught in a severe winter storm and became disoriented and lost. Unable to find the safety of the Fort, they were forced to spend the night in the storm. When they were found the next morning, Lt. Morgan had died from exposure and Webster, though still alive, had frozen feet. Dr. Wheaton was of the opinion that Webster would probably need an amputation but wanted to delay the operation. He apparently decided that the operation could wait until he returned from his holiday to Kaukauna. While Dr. Wheaton was absent, his brother, whose only training in surgery was limited reading and observing his older sibling, was watching the patient. He observation convinced him that an operation was needed immediately or Webster would die the very same night. He asked the post commander's permission to amputate the frozen limbs. The commander agreed, and the eighteen- year-old man proceeded to complete the amputation on Webster and probably saved his life. When Dr. Wheaton finally returned , Webster was on his way to recovery and lived for many years. [6]

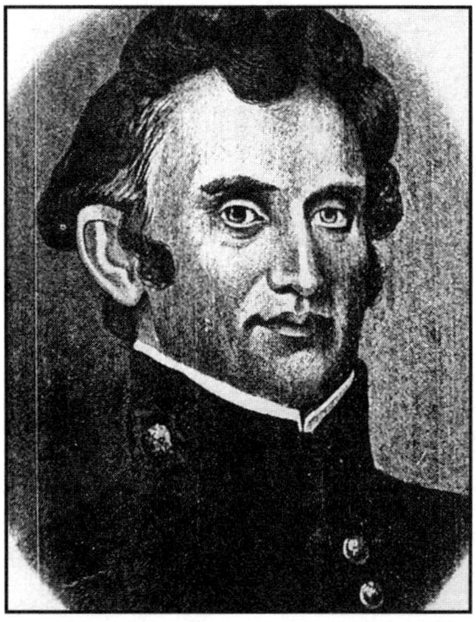

Dr. William Beaumont 1785 - 1853
Reprinted from *Wisconsin Magazine of History*, Vol. IV, 3, March 1921 published by Wisconsin State Historical Society.

Dr. William Beaumont succeeded Dr. Wheaton in 1826. Dr. Beaumont, as many early nineteenth century physicians, did not attend any of the medical schools in existence. He received his training through reading medical books and apprenticing himself to Dr. Benjamin Chandler, of St. Albans, Vermont. He was able to pass a certifying exam given by the Third Medical Society of Vermont and claim the title of MD. Soon afterward, Dr. Beaumont began his military service as a surgeon's mate. Much of his surgical experience was gained on the battlefield near Plattsburg, New York, treating the wounded and sick during the War of 1812 . He resigned from the service after the war and entered private practice before rejoining the army in 1820 and being sent to Fort Mackinac

Dr. Beaumont began his famous digestive experiments on Alexis St. Martin at Fort Mackinac. The observations and experiments were on hold during Dr. Beaumont's duty at Fort Howard. Unfortunately, these experiments were not to continue until Beaumont was transferred to Prairie Du Chien in 1828. St. Martin, whose gunshot wound had healed with an opening into his stomach allowing gastric juice to be removed and experimental substances inserted, eluded the doctor who was eager to do further testing. St. Martin was eventually brought back to Fort Crawford by Dr. Beaumont and more experiments carried on utilizing the gastric cutaneous fistula. Dr. Beaumont's reputation as a physician and scientist had preceded his appearance in Green Bay. He had already sent the initial experiments on the effects of gastric juice for publication. Already a respected physician, Dr. Beaumont, however, was not without controversy. [7]

While stationed at Fort Mackinac, Dr. Beaumont maintained a garden for raising vegetables, greens, and herbs, which he deemed important for the health of the troops. He had learned the use of plants for healing from his apprenticeship in Vermont. In addition to the medicinal plants, he grew hops to make beer to reduce the troops' dependency on whisky. Each soldier was issued a whisky ration as part of his compensation. (It was not until 1830 that the whisky ration was discontinued and the whisky turned over to the control of the medical department.). The Indian agent on Mackinac, Colonel George Boyd, asked to construct a building on the garden site next to the hospital. (Colonel Boyd was married to the sister-in-law of President John Q. Adams.) Approval for the building was denied by Captain Ben K. Pierce, but he was overruled by General Macomb. Beaumont protested to the Chief Army Surgeon, Dr. Lovell. Fortunately, Dr. Lovell, who had served with Beaumont during the War of 1812 was also very concerned with providing vegetables and a healthy diet for the troops. The welfare of the troops won out, and Dr. Beaumont was allowed to keep his garden. [8]

In 1825 Dr. Beaumont was transferred to Fort Niagara in New York. While there, Lieutenant Edmund B. Griswald had reported to the hospital because of presumed illness. Two of his fellow officers felt he was not performing his duties and should report to the surgeon for evaluation. After examination and standard treatment including bleeding, Dr. Beaumont ultimately thought Lieutenant Griswald was fit for duty. Griswald did not agree. Finding no signs of illness, Beaumont thought Griswald was malingering and decided to test his theory by giving the Lieutenant a dose of medication (Calomel and tartar emetic) that would ordinarily produce soreness and blisters in the mouth. Observing no symptoms over twenty-four hours, Dr. Beaumont surmised that the Lt. Griswald did not take the medication. Dr. Beaumont concluded Lt. Griswald did not take the prescribed medication because he was never ill and thus there was substantial evidence he was malingering. Lt. Griswald was reported to the commander, court martialed, and sentenced to be dismissed from service. Because the officers who originally initiated the complaint of neglect of duty later reversed themselves and now backed their fellow officer, the court martial decision was overturned, but not before the case eventually got all the way to President Adams who rebuked Beaumont for the deceptive practice of using medication without cause. [9]

Dr. T. S. Bryant was present at Fort Howard in 1827. He and Beaumont were involved in another dispute. Dr. Byrant had put a splint on a soldier's leg for treatment of a fracture. The diagnosis was questioned. Dr. Beaumont did not concur in the diagnosis and the splint removed. Medical treatment cured the leg pain and the soldier returned to duty. Dr. Bryant was charged with malpractice. The chief witness against Byrant was Dr. Beaumont. Again the President of the United States, John Q. Adams, intervened, and the charges were dropped. [10]

Despite these controversies, Dr. Beaumont was well respected by the community. In addition to his military duties, he was called upon to minister to the settlers and Indians. He was the first in the territory to administer vaccinations for smallpox. While at Fort Mackinac and again at Fort Howard, he asked the Army Surgeon's office to send a smallpox scab to use for vaccine. The practice was to incubate the scab in warm water and place the liquid on the skin after a cut was made to produce bleeding. Not sure if the first scab that arrived was effective after the long arduous journey from the East, he petitioned Dr. Lovell to send two more scabs. Dr. Lovell, wanting to be sure the scabs were being utilized correctly by his controversial friend, sent along instructions for the soon to be immortalized scientist. [11]

The Army's inspection report in 1828 noted that the Fort Howard hospital was in "poor condition and entirely destitute of means of comfort save medicines." The building was noted to "need some repairs and alterations to render it secure against rain and more convenient." Dr. Beaumont complained that the surgical instruments were not fit for use. He advocated each surgeon be issued a set and be responsible for its maintenance. The inspector went on to commend Dr. Beaumont. "Assistant Surgeon William Beaumont acts with an exclusive eye to the comfort of the sick." The inspector also thought it appropriate to remark on the doctors' medical library. He noted the library contained ***The Treatise on Gonorrhea Virulents and Leus***, Benjamin Bell, 1814; ***Lectures on Principles and Practices of Surgery***, Sir Astley Paston Cooper, 1825; ***Acute and Chronic Diseases***, Thomas Syndenham, 1809; ***Diseases of the Army***, Sir John Pringle,1810; and ***Modern Practice of Physic***, Robert Thomas, 1817. The inspector further noted: " The best medical journals and most approved treatises on mineralogy and botany are much wanted at all frontier posts... to enable them to report with confidence and correctly upon the mineralogical and botanical wealth of their several districts." [12]

Dr. Beaumont exhibited a compassion for the welfare of the troops. He was not afraid of the consequences of expressing his views. He believed the environment and weather conditions were important factors in health and disease. Before leaving Fort Howard, he wrote a letter to the incoming surgeon, Dr. Lyman Foot, concerning the hazards to which the troops were exposed when gathering hay for the post livestock . Dr. Beaumont attributed the soldiers' diseased swollen feet to the swampy conditions, presence of poisonous reptiles, and poisonous roots surrounding the Fort. He and Dr. Richard Satterlee, assistant surgeon at that time, both advocated civilian procurement of the cattle feed. Not long afterward a civilian contract was executed and the soldiers relieved of gathering hay. [13]

Dr. Beaumont was present during the Winnebago unrest and hostilities of 1824-1827. Major Whistler, commander of Fort Howard, used a display of military force to obtain Chief Red Bird's surrender without loss of life. However, before leaving Green Bay, Dr. Beaumont was to charge Major Whistler with drunkenness on duty, a serious offense. No action was taken, and surprisingly, Dr. Beaumont continued his career without repercussions. [14]

The Army had reduced the total number of medical officers to fifty-three in 1821 following the conclusion of the War of 1812. There were eight surgeons and forty-eight assistant surgeons allotted for all the Army posts. Dr. Beaumont was one of only eight surgeons in the Army in 1828. The rest were assistant surgeons. Being an Army doctor was not a healthy occupation in the early nineteenth century. Between 1821 and 1832, six frontier doctors died, Dr. Madison was shot, and the other five died of illness. [15]

Dr. Worrell was assigned to Fort Howard in 1828. He was described as a bachelor who was very reserved and did not make friends easily. Dr. Lyman Foot, a graduate of Yale Medical School entered the Army in 1819 and was assigned to Fort Howard in 1828, also. "He made friends readily and kept a large civilian practice. Settlers who had relied on various home remedies often called him. He also was respected because of his social graces." [16] The army inspector noted Dr. Foot "has managed the medical department with much care and attention. Sick list is long this summer but no contagious disease, most cases are accidental wounds or diseases brought on by dissipated habits." [17]

1829 marked the arrival of the first civilian physician in Wisconsin. Dr. David Ward began his practice in Green Bay but also was hired as an acting assistant surgeon at Fort Howard. It was not unusual to employ civilians to staff the military medical facilities. There was a need for more medical personnel because Congress had provided funds in 1827 to construct a military road from Fort Howard to Fort Winnebago, near Portage, Wisconsin. Three years later, funds were appropriated to continue the road to Fort Crawford in Prairie Du Chien. The soldiers were employed to build the road. A physician usually accompanied the troops to treat the wounds and illnesses that frequently occurred.

The frontier doctor depended upon his senses for diagnosis. The character of the pulse and appearance of the tongue were used as clues to the diagnosis and prognosis. Unfortunately, there was little beyond diagnosis that was to the benefit to the patient. The troops were subject to the same maladies as the settlers. Cholera, small pox, typhoid fever, influenza, dysentery, erysipelas, tuberculosis, and venereal disease were common. Malaria, although common in the Midwest, was not prevalent at Fort Howard prior to 1828. Injuries and accidents were common problems. Surgery was limited to amputations, repairing ruptures, draining of abscesses, trepanning, and removing superficial cancers.

An epidemic of cholera occurred in Green Bay in 1832 and again in 1834. The cholera epidemic was probably brought to Wisconsin by the military. General Winfield Scott and troops traveled from Buffalo, New York, to Fort Crawford, Wisconsin, in hopes of ending the Black Hawk Indian uprising. General Scott arrived after the fighting, but severe outbreaks of cholera occurred wherever he camped. The disease spread rapidly to the settlement at Green Bay. Many died from the illness. Father Vanden Broek attended the sick and dying at Green Bay. During the height of the epidemic, the deaths were so frequent that burial of four or five at once was necessary. There were so few healthy settlers that the priest and nuns had to help with burials.

The Winnebago Indians were devastated by an outbreak of smallpox in 1832-1834. Nearly one fourth of the tribe died. The remaining Indians actually fled their camp because of the severity of the outbreak. Apparently, neither smallpox nor cholera reached epidemic proportions among the troops at Fort Howard.

Treatment for infectious diseases were limited. The humoral theory of disease was still widely accepted. This theory attributed sickness to an imbalance of the four basic humors: blood, phlegm, black bile, and yellow bile. Other theories projected a chemical imbalance as the cause of disease. Dr. Benjamin Rush, prominent American physician, in 1800 proposed three factors for the cause of fevers. A predisposing debility, an internal or external influence, and a convulsive excitement in the walls of the blood vessels were common to all diseases. He advised reducing the convulsive excitement of the blood vessels. This meant actively and aggressively removing the offending agent or exciting cause. Most frontier doctors treated fever with bleeding, vomiting, and purging to rid the body of the offending agents. Blistering was also used to create a counter illness in the hopes that deleterious humors would leave the patient. Blistering involved use of ground cantharides (dried beetles) that produced a skin burn. Remedies frequently differed between doctors and were usually based upon their formal education but more often upon their experience in the field. Many doctors also used the native herbs that grew in the territory. Prevailing practice accepted the belief that the more aggressive the approach, the better. The aggressive, debilitating treatments often resulted in death. The disastrous mortality statistics for illness did little to alter the practice. The patients were to be admired for their courage during the treatment.

The army inspector's report concerning Fort Howard in September 1833 noted: "eleven in hospital, most remittent fever. This post and the country immediately about it are becoming more unhealthy every year, and cases of fever do now occur of a character such as formerly did not make their appearance. This is ascribable to the draining of the marshes in the rear of the fort, by which a large surface of vegetable matter in a state of decomposition is left exposed and free to emit its poisonous effluvia." [18]

Dr. Daniel Drake, prominent educator, scientist, and physician of the first half of the nineteenth century, compiled a large volume of data to explain the types and treatment of "autumnal fever." He thought the cause may have been due to a combination of noxious gas from the decaying soil and an animal vector source but did not have definitive proof of either. In Drake's book, Dr. David Ward is given credit for describing the extensive marshes surrounding Fort Howard. Dr. Drake concluded that the higher elevation and warmer climate of Fort Winnebago at Portage, compared to Fort Howard terrain, accounted for the lower incidence of autumnal fever from the noxious influence.

Treatment of autumnal fever was related to the stages of fever. During the initial excitatory stage, bleeding and purging were advocated. Curative medications included Chinchona bark, stimulants, and tonics. Capsicum, ammonia, gentian columba, and carbonate of iron were suggested by Drake.

Dr. Richard S. Satterlee returned to Fort Howard as surgeon in September 1933. Dr. C. A. Finley served briefly between 1830 and 1831. Dr. Satterlee graduated from the College of Physicians and Surgeons of the Western District of New York and joined the Army in 1822. His previous service at Fort Howard had been as assistant surgeon. Young Dr. Satterlee made a very favorable impression on the population of Green Bay. He and his wife were described as a very handsome couple. A devout man, Dr.

Satterlee was involved in organizing the first Presbyterian church in Wisconsin and participated in the Temperance Society in Green Bay.

It was during the tenure of Dr. Satterlee that the hospital was rebuilt. The army inspector's report noted the poor condition of the hospital in 1834. "Medicines and stores sufficient. Location not as healthy as used to be. Eighteen in hospital, twenty-four sick with rheumatism, catarrah, ophthalmia. Only one sick ward in hospital, small and poor ventilation, hot in summer. Only space for ten cots, some need placed on floor. House in bad repair, roof not tight enough to keep out rain. In 1826 condemned hospital as unsuitable and every visit reported against it." [19]

The new hospital was built soon afterward in the same location outside the walls of the fort. The plans were drawn by Dr. Satterlee. The hospital had two wards for eight patients each but was capable of handling forty-four patients if necessary. Included in the layout was a kitchen, doctor's office, and mess. This hospital has been restored and is presently located at Heritage Hill State Park.

The Quarterly Report of the Sick and Wounded from December 1834 was completed by Dr. Satterlee. Seventy-nine soldiers were listed as sick or wounded. There were nineteen ill with influenza, nine catarrh, five lumbago, five dyspepsia, six wounds, three gonorrhea, three syphilis, four rheumatism, four diarrhea and six ophthalmia. Dr. Satterlee deemed it appropriate to comment on the death of one soldier under his care.

Since the Cholera Morbus disappearance, Influenza has prevailed to some extent in the garrison, it exhibited symptoms of different in some degree from common catarrh. I have in the reports separated the cases. The case that terminated in the death reported excited symptoms of great inflammation of the facial & glands of the throat, though not an extraordinary excitement of the pulse. I have found it necessary to let blood in some cases, but not generally. Emetics have also in some cases proved salutary. The treatment that has succeeded best in my hands consists in cathartics, sudorifics, low diet, gargling the throat in peppered vinegar and salt, and expectorants. As an expectorant I have used a preparation of gum ammoniac with honey and paregoric, with advantage. I deem it not improper to remark that this is the first death that has occurred from disease while I have been stationed since I have been in the Army. [20]

Dr. Satterlee described a particularly prolonged course of treatment of a private who died on Christmas Day 1836, after two months of intensive care.

The man who died on the twenty-fifth was rather an uncommon case, only, however, from the fact, that he continued to do his duty as a labourer on the road, and did not even ask advice for the affection of the lungs but presented himself to Doctor

Wright (who was with the working party) with a slight wound of the leg. But on examination a day or two after he found him labouring under chronic pneumonitis and apparently of several months standing. He treated him by extensive counter irritation over the left lung, the presumed site of the lesion, with expectorants, minute doses of antimony, and occasional doses of opiates to check the colliquative diarrhea which had already become quite troublesome. He used no depletion for he had no operatives for cupping. He returned to the Garrison on the first of Nov, when he came under my charge in Hospital.

He was tall, slim, very narrow chest, harassed with cough difficulty of breathing. Hestick paravision in afternoon, night sweats and profuse diarrhea, pulse considerably accelarated and rather hard. He was bled from the arm which he bore well and cupped over the region of the pain, an effort was made to control the circulation by Antimony, but this he could not tolerate for it increased the diarrhea, to stop which opiates were given, this for a day or two seemed to produce good effect but soon failed. Various prescriptions were tried, a decoction of Rhubarb with Tinc Opium and dark refined sugar seemed for a time to have a good effect, and then Muriatic Acid with Opium was tried ineffectively, but these two last prescriptions combined seemed more beneficial than any other. Trial was also made of the Digitalis (but this was entirely inadviseable it reproduced the diarrhea which had been partially checked and brought on immediate and alarming prostration) With tartar emetic plaster over the left breast: nothing however seemed to arrest the rapid march of the disease which terminated in Phthisis Pulmonalis and he died as before stated on the twenty-fifth of December 1836. [21]

Dr. J. J. Wright was assigned to Fort Howard 1835-1837. He had graduated from University of Pennsylvania in 1826 and joined the Army in 1833. "A man of conspicuous tact and courtesy, he had a high sense of justice and honor and possessed a high concept of the obligations of the soldier." [22] Dr. Philip Maxwell also was present for a brief period in 1837.

The quarterly report signed by Dr. Satterlee for the three months ending March 1837, noted the usually increased incidence of catarrh and rheumatism during the winter. Thirty soldiers had reported sick with catarrh. They were treated with "cathartics and diaphoretics: the lancet has sometimes been required, but not generally." Fifteen were diagnosed with rheumatism. "The latter disease has been more intractable, as it usually is particularly here; it has been treated by bleeding, local and general, cathartics, and after the inflammatory action has begun to subside, pispastics and Colchicum Autumnale continued until it acts upon the bowels smartly, has been found very efficacious, and after this guaiacum and Dovers powder has been successfully used." [23]

Dr. Ward had gone back East and returned in 1834 with a bride. His advertisement appeared in the Green Bay Intelligencer in January 1834. "D. Ward Physician and Surgeon Continues the practice of Medicine in Navarino and its vicinity. He has taken an office in the front part of the building occupied by the Green Bay Intelligencer, where he will always be ready, and happy to attend any calls in his profession." Three months later, in March 1834, Dr. Ward moved his office to the corner of Washington and Main, site of Mr. Whitney's Tavern house. In 1847, Dr. David Ward was an original member of the State Medical Society of Wisconsin.

Dr. George Armstrong settled in Green Bay about 1835. Dr. Armstrong, a civilian, also was temporarily employed by the military. Mrs. Elizabeth Baird apparently preferred the latter doctor over Dr. Ward. The first non-military physicians had to supplement their incomes from the practice of medicine just as the military physicians were eager to have a civilian practice for extra income. Fees in the 1830's were fifty cents for a daytime house call and seventy cents for a night call. The 1830 census of Brown County recorded 1263 of which two hundred twenty one were soldiers. The difficulty in collecting fees and the sparse population forced the civilian physician to be adaptable. As late as 1849, Dr. A. B.Williams of De Pere was hunting to feed his family.

Dr. Stoddard Judd came to Green Bay from a practice in the East in 1841. He was a graduate of Albany Medical College in 1819. A delegate to the Wisconsin constitutional conventions, he was described as "a man of decided ability and possessed of great energy of character." He left Green in 1845 to practice in southern Wisconsin. [24]

The military physician era ended in 1851 with Dr. Richard Simpson. Fort Howard was almost emptied of troops after 1841. Indian hostilities ended with the surrender of Black Hawk and there was little need for a military presence. The opportunity for civilian doctors was much improved. The population had doubled between 1832 and 1836 and was continuing to grow. The practice of medicine had not changed dramatically in Wisconsin and Brown County since the first Army doctor arrived. In 1847, the accepted practice of medicine still consisted of bleeding, purging, vomiting, injections, blistering, poultices, and symptomatic fever therapy. Surgery was limited to amputations, trepanning, repairing cuts and superficial surgery. Retail stores sold drugs and devices to treat most any disease. *The Green Bay Advocate* of 1849 had detailed ads for liquid preparations, magnets, and garments that would help the sickest recover from a variety of ailments.

Notes to Chapter 1

1. Kavasch, E., Baar, Karen, *American Indian Healing Arts*, Bantam Books, 1999.
2. Poquette, Moses, The Wisconsin Winnebago Remedies, *Wisconsin Historical Collections*, vol. 12 pg. 424.
3. Thomas, G. Capt., Narrative, *Wisconsin Historical Collections*, vol. 10, pg. 104-5.
4. Colonel Childs Recollections Since 1826, *Wisconsin Historical Collections* vol. 4 pg. 164.
5. *War Department Army File*, Record Group 94, 108, 1812-1826 and 1830-1845. Inspections of Fort Howard Hospital on microfilm located at Brown County Library, Green Bay, Wisconsin.
6. Ellis, Albert G. Recollections, *Wisconsin Historical Collections*, vol. 7 pg. 259.
7. Horseman, Reginald, Frontier Doctor: *William Beaumont, America's First Great Scientist*, University Missouri Press, 1996.
8. Nelson, Rodney B., *Beaumont*, Grant House Press, 1990.
9. ibid.
10. ibid.
11. ibid.
12. Croghan, Colonel George, *U.S. Army Official Reports* 1826-1845, University of Oklahoma Press.
13. *Returns From U.S. Military Posts* 1818-1851, National Archives, USA Microfilm 488- 489, Brown County,Wisconsin Library.
14. See note 7.
15. See note 8.
16. Baird, Elizabeth T., *Memoirs*, Heritage Hill Foundation 1998.
17. *Green Bay Historical Bulletin*, September- October, 1928, vol. 4 no. 5.
18. See note 12.
19. See note 12.
20. *U.S. Adjuvent General Quarterly Returns of Sick and Wounded*, Fort Howard, Wisconsin 1834-1837, Brown County Library Wisconsin, microfilm.
21. ibid.
22. Tenney, H.A., Atwood, Dave, *Memorial Record of The Fathers Of Wisconsin*, pg. 107-8, 1880.
23. See note 20.
24. ibid.

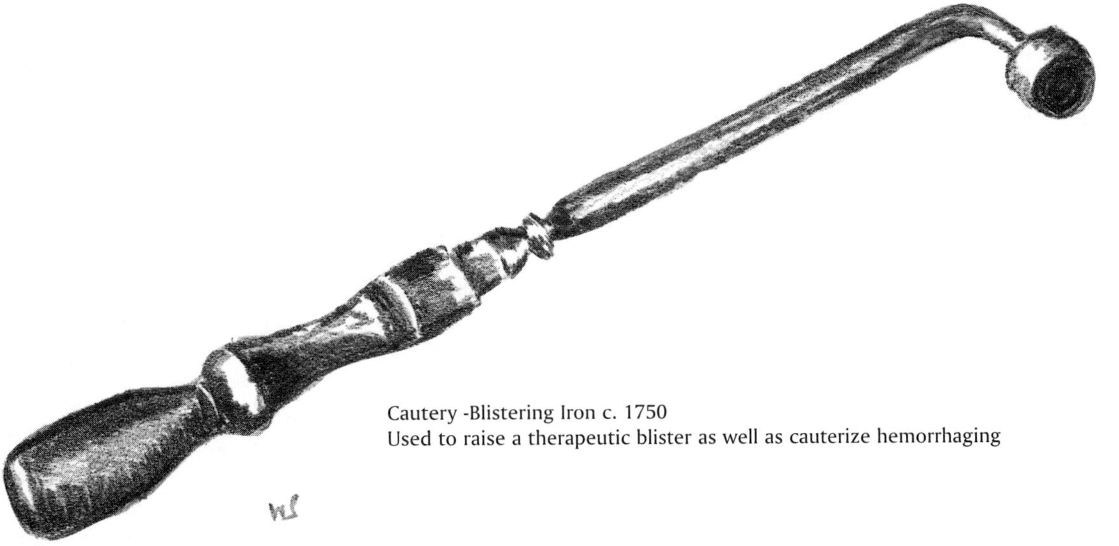

Cautery -Blistering Iron c. 1750
Used to raise a therapeutic blister as well as cauterize hemorrhaging

Chapter 2

Cadle Home

The closing of the Fort Howard Hospital in 1852 ended the era of military medicine in Green Bay. The threat of Indian hostilities had subsided and the need for a military garrison in northeast Wisconsin was no longer present. Fur trading as an industry was being replaced by logging and lumber mills. Farming, shipping, and related services provided the newly arrived with work. The population of the territory had grown by the westward movement of Americans and immigrants from abroad. The census of 1850 indicated 6,215 residents of Brown County, compared to 1,500 including 300 soldiers in 1830.

Wisconsin was organized as a territory in 1836 and in 1848 received statehood. During this time the southern section of the state had grown more rapidly than Brown County, and consequently, many more physicians began medical practice in that region of the new state. In the period between the phase out of Fort Howard and the Civil War, records indicated only six new physicians began practices in Brown County.

Dr. Louis Carabin Sr. arrived in 1846. He practiced in Green Bay and West De Pere until his death in 1864. He apparently built the first house in West De Pere. Not much else is known of his work. The first physician in De Pere was Dr. A. B. Williams. He practiced from 1847 until precisely 10 a.m. on February 28, 1875. His wife recalled the struggle to make a living in medicine during his early years of practice. Initially, few patients came to see Dr. Williams. For weeks the family would live on fish and game caught by the doctor as there were few cases of sickness among the eleven families nearby. Eventually, he became very successful and was able to establish a large practice which necessitated a partner. He literally practiced until his dying day. According to Dr. Williams' wife, on the day of his death, he wrote a prescription at 10 a.m. and by 1 p.m. he was gone! [1]

Dr. C. E. Crane and Dr. Israel Green came to Green Bay in 1849. Dr. Green was born in New York January 26,1792 and received his MD degree in 1816 from the New York College of Physicians and Surgeons. He continued to practice medicine until the age of ninety-four and died in 1881 at the age of ninety-nine. [2]

Dr. Charles E. Crane was educated in the Norwalk, Ohio school system and read medicine at Western Reserve College. He came directly to Green Bay to begin practice with Dr. Carabin. Dr. Crane enlisted in the 5th Wisconsin Infantry Regiment in 1861 and participated in the second Battle of Bull Run, Chancelorsville, Fredericksburg, and

Rappahonek Bridge. After returning from the war, he became active in organizing the Brown County Medical Society and served as its president from 1868 to 1880. In addition to his medical practice, he also served on the school board for six years and was mayor of Green Bay for five years, 1874-75 and 1877-79. [3]

The Civil War had an impact on medicine in Brown County. The treatment of battlefield injuries and illnesses of the troops during the war began to change the practice of medicine in Brown County. Bleeding, purging, vomiting, although still practiced, were less of the norm. Old practices, however, were hard to change. The head of the Union Army Medical Corp was removed from office early in the Civil War because he tried to improve command efficiency through an overhaul of the organization of the Union Army Medical Corp and to update therapy of illness by removing unproved remedies such as calomel and tartar emetic from the surgeon's supply of drugs. Surgical care was evolving with the experience. The use of carbolic acid, iodine, and turpentine for wounds recognized a concern for antisepsis during surgery. Chloroform and ether were available in some locations in the United States and may have been used for surgery. Technical skills of surgeons were honed by a sometimes overwhelming experience on the wounded. Unfortunately, many of the soldiers were casualties of disease during the war. The importance of sanitation of the camps was recognized as a contribution to the high rate of morbidity and mortality among the troops. Outbreaks of typhoid, dysentery, and respiratory ailments were thought to be directly related to overcrowding and contaminated water. [4] The war undoubtedly played a major role in the lives of military surgeons who returned to the civilian practice of medicine in Brown County. Many of the surgeons who served were to provide strong leadership locally and statewide.

Dr. Cooper Ayres began practice in 1850 but was interrupted to serve as a Union Army surgeon for the 7th Infantry Regiment, 1861 to 1864. Soon after beginning practice in Green Bay he became active in the State Medical Society. Dr. David Ward, as mentioned previously, was one of the organizers and a member of the Society in 1847. The Society was reorganized in 1854 and Dr. Cooper was elected first vice-president. The following year he was chosen to give a paper on ascites (intra-abdominal fluid) to the Society. The presentations were an attempt by the Society to educate members in the new and unusual. The case reports did not involve any rigorous scientific examination but each case was discussed and criticized by fellow members. There were only a few attendees at the state meeting. Sixteen members were present in 1857 when Dr. Ayres was elected president of the State Medical Society. He received a plurality of five votes with one abstention. Total membership was fifty statewide. He was also appointed a delegate to the American Medical Association. Dr. Ayres continued practice in Green Bay until the early 1870s. [5]

De Pere was the site chosen by Dr. James T. Reeve, a graduate of Jefferson Medical College, to begin medical practice in 1856. He moved to Green Bay in 1859 before enlisting and receiving an appointment as assistant surgeon to the 10th Infantry Regiment. He attained the rank of brigade surgeon and acting medical director of the 1st division 14th Army Corp. He was captured by the Confederates at Chickamauga Creek because he felt obliged to stay with the wounded when the Union Army was forced to abandon his hospital. He was held prisoner for nine weeks before being released. After the war he started a practice in Appleton. In 1875, Dr. Reeve was elected president of the State Medical Society. [6]

Very few European trained physicians settled in Green Bay. One of the first was Henry Rhode. He was born in Hanover, Germany and received his MD from the University of Goettingen in 1850. After serving in the Russian Army until 1854, he first settled in Toledo, Ohio but left following the deaths of his father, mother, and two sisters during one of the cholera epidemics. He practiced until about 1881. Dr. Henry Pearce arrived in 1860 from London, England where he trained as a homeopathic physician. He worked in Green Bay for fifteen years. His obituary appeared in the *Green Bay Advocate* of May 28, 1875. The comment in the obituary reflected the high regard many of the physicians of the day enjoyed. “We fear that he has left his family in scarcely comfortable circumstances due to his generous ways and disinclination to collect his fees. Cheery greetings, his honest examples, his wide charity and generosity, his good counsels, his faithful friendships, and boundless ingathering of all that constituted a man, husband, father, citizen, and neighbor and a Christian gentleman will survive the grief of this day.” [7]

Dr. Andrew Munroe immigrated from Scotland to practice in Green Bay. Dr. P. Marchand, a French physician also came after the Civil War ended. Both were to practice faithfully into the 1880s.

Dr. G. A. Lamb, who was an assistant surgeon with the 40th Wisconsin Regiment, left the army to settle in Green Bay in 1864. Dr. H. O. Crane (no relation to C. E. Crane) also took part in the Civil War as a surgeon. He received his MD from Western Reserve College in 1848 and was an assistant surgeon for the 3rd Wisconsin volunteers. After discharge he was appointed examining surgeon for the 5th Wisconsin Congressional District. Statistics from his work as an examining physician noted a very high rate of rejection. Forty-eight out of every 1,000 recruits were turned down because of hernia and twelve out of every 1,000 recruits were rejected because of fracture or dislocation.

Dr. A. H. Van Norstrand moved to Green Bay From Madison, Wisconsin in 1868. He had been Superintendent of the Madison State Hospital. His Civil War experience was with the 4th Wisconsin Regiment. He did not open a clinical practice in Green Bay but remained active in the Medical Society. Eventually, his residence was sold to the Sisters of the Third Order of St. Francis for a hospital.

Twenty physicians were in Green Bay and De Pere by 1872. In addition to those already mentioned, Drs. W. W. Goff, H. Elderkin, W. H. Bartran, Mary Camm, Nanscawen, and Peake practiced in Green Bay and Drs. Fisk, Emery, Jackson, Carscadden, Crocker, and Pitcher were in De Pere.

Homeopathic, osteopathic and eclectic herbal practitioners established a presence in Wisconsin after the Civil War. Drs. Nanscawen and Camm were homeopaths. Mary Camm was probably the first woman physician to practice in Brown County. Little is recorded about her practice. Her daughter married Dr. Wellington B. Coffeen, also a homeopathic physician. Mary Camm died at age fifty-five. "She was held in loving and kindly remembrance for her many acts of charity and devotion to the sick and afflicted." [8] Apparently homeopathy was readily accepted by the patients.

Another homeopathic physician, Dr. Austin F. Olmsted began practice in Green Bay in 1874 after graduating from Cleveland Homeopathic College. Born in 1843, his family moved to Wisconsin in 1850. Four years later, his father died. At age fifteen, Austin F. Olmsted quit school to help work the farm. Eventually, after attending Lawerence College for two years, he decided to go to Cleveland, Ohio Homeopathic College, graduating in 1874. Dr. Olmsted was recognized as an obstetrician. Dr. W. H. Squire joined him in practice for a few years and then in 1902, Dr. Olmsted's son, Dr. Austin O. Olmsted returned to practice medicine in Green Bay. Like his father, "he was a firm believer in the principles of homeopathy and has always practiced medicine according to these principles." [9]

Dr. William H. Bartran was superintendent of schools for Fort Howard and later served as mayor of Fort Howard in 1891. He was also a state representative from 1873-1874. A soldier in the Civil War, he was wounded at the Battle of Bull Run. After the war he graduated from the University Michigan College at Ann Arbor. He established an office at the corner of Broadway and Main Street in Fort Howard in 1869. His specialty was surgery. [10]

The Peshtigo fire of 1871 left many people homeless, poor, and suffering. Drs. Rhode, Elderkin, Munro, and Fisk set out early on the evening of the fire to treat the sick and injured. Public places and halls were filled with the ill and destitute as a result of the fire. The old Turners Hall, under the supervision of Dr. H.O. Crane was designated as a relief hospital. About $90,000 was raised to provide help to the ill and poor. The Women's Aid Society of Christ Episcopal Church received a portion of that sum to establish a hospital. Articles of incorporation were adopted in May 1872 for the purpose of "erecting, establishing, and maintaining a home and hospital, for the education and maintenance of orphan children, for the care and relief of sick, infirm, needy, destitute or homeless persons, for the care and support of aged and infirm clergymen, or for any or all of these or such other charitable purposes as this corporation may, from time to time carry into execution." [11] It was called Cadle Home. The building was named after Rev. Cadle, a missionary to the area. It was located at the southwest corner of Pine and Madison streets, to the rear of Christ Church. Completed in 1874, it was in use for about eight years. Drs. Green and Pearce were members of the original board. The building was sixty-six by fifty-four feet and was divided into twenty-two rooms. There were never more than five or six patients at one time. This was Green Bay's first civilian hospital. The building lacked accommodations for aseptic techniques, and no contagious diseases were admitted. Since there were no trained nurses in the area, three matrons administered to the patients. Mrs. Couley, Mrs. Kate Hume, and Mrs. Robinson were in charge. Dr. B. C. Brett was one of the first to publicly volunteer his services without charge to the patients.

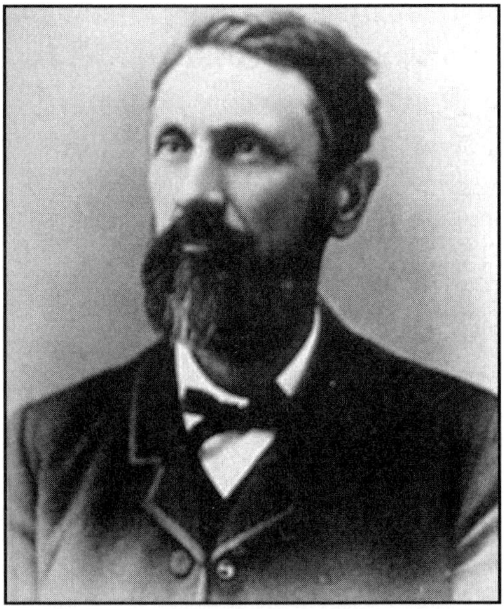

Dr. Benjamin C. Brett
1833 - 1931
Photo courtesy of
Grand Army Publishing Co. 1888

Dr. Benjamin C. Brett transferred his medical practice from Brodhead, Wisconsin to Green Bay in 1872. Dr. Brett received his education at Bowdoin College and then served a preceptorship with a country doctor. Texts during the preceptorship included ***Wilson's Anatomy***, ***Wood's Practice***, ***United States Dispensatory***, ***Druit's Surgery***, and ***Churchill's Midwifery***. He read medicine for three years and had two course of lectures, three months each, before graduating from Dartmouth College Medical Department in 1860 with a medical degree. He then took a position with a New York Dispensory because he felt "ill prepared to practice." Dr. Brett served in the 21st Wisconsin Infantry Regiment during the Civil War. He was captured by the Confederates at the Battle of Murfreesboro and later released. He had been in charge of as many as five hundred sick and wounded. Dr. Brett noted that the Army doctors had few medicines available for the sick. His bag contained "Epsom salts, blue mass, quinine (which the men usually threw away before reaching quarters), morphine, calomel, and Dover's powder." [12]

Active in preventive health, a leader in the medical community, and respected physician, Dr. Brett retired in 1913 at the age of eighty-six. He was the municipal health officer for Green Bay for nineteen years. A biographical sketch in *Men Who are Making Green Bay* published in 1897 states, "During the long period of his residence in Green Bay, Dr. Brett has been intelligently active and influential touching all things affecting the sanitary conditions of the city. He has been a trusted advisor of the municipal government in matters relating to sanitary legislation, and his recommendations, which have been invariably good, have in many cases been made part of the laws and ordinances of Green Bay."

His peers elected him president of the Wisconsin State Medical Society in 1894. In his presidential address to the Society in 1894, he urged the members to act on several contemporary issues. The public needed protection from charlatans and non-regular physicians. Patent medicines needed labeling as to the ingredients; burial permits were necessary to document the cause of death and thus prevent the public health hazard of potential unrecognized epidemics of disease; expert medical witnesses should be selected by judges to avoid the potential of unqualified and untruthful testimony; and physicians need training in economics to be sure they have income as patients tended to pay the MD last. [13] Some of these same issues face today's doctors.

He was also instrumental in reorganizing the Brown County Medical Society in 1903 and served as the first president.

1883 saw the arrival of Dr. Hans Beck from Germany. Prior to receiving his medical degree from Rush Medical College, he was a pharmacist. In addition to his practice, he was a member of the US Board of Pension examiners and a member of the Green Bay Board of School Commissioners. [14] A brief article appeared in the *Green Bay Advocate* of May 28, 1875. "Doctor Hans Beck and Andrew Munroe assisted by A. O. Duchateau removed an encysted abscess from the shoulder of Mr. Jensen of Marinette at the US Hotel in Green Bay. They also removed some dead bone." There was no public hospital in Brown County.

Notes to Chapter 2

1. French, Bella, *History of Brown County, American Sketchbook*, Memories of De Pere, pg. 132. Mrs. A. B. Williams recounts the difficulty her husband had in beginning a medical practice.
2. *Green Bay Advocate*, Obituary of Dr. Israel Green August 8, 1886.
3. *Commemorative Biographical Record of the Counties of Brown, Kewaunee, and Door, Wisconsin*, J. H. Beerr and Co., Chicago, IL 1895.
4. Duffy, John, *Humors to Medical Science*, University IL Press, 1993.
5. *Transactions of the Wisconsin State Medical Society*, 1842-1873, University of Wisconsin Medical

Library, Madison, Wisconsin.

6. *United States Biographical Dictionary*.
7. *Green Bay Advocate*, Obituary of Dr. Henry Pearce, May 28, 1875.
8. See note 3.
9. Martin, Deborah Beaumont. *History of Brown County, Past and Present*, S. J. Clark Co. Chicago, 1913.
10. ibid.
11. Cadle Home and Hospital, Records of the Christ Episcopal Church, Green Bay, 1829-1961, University of Wisconsin Green Bay Historical Collection.
12. Manuscript of Dr. Benjamin C. Brett, 1923, University of Wisconsin Green Bay Historical Collection. Dr. Brett recorded his recollection of the Cadle Home and other incidents of his life as a practitioner.
13. *Transactions of the State Medical Society*, President's address to the society, 1894, University of Wisconsin Medical Library, Madison, Wisconsin.
14. *Men Who Are Making Green Bay*, Gazette Publishing Co. 1897.

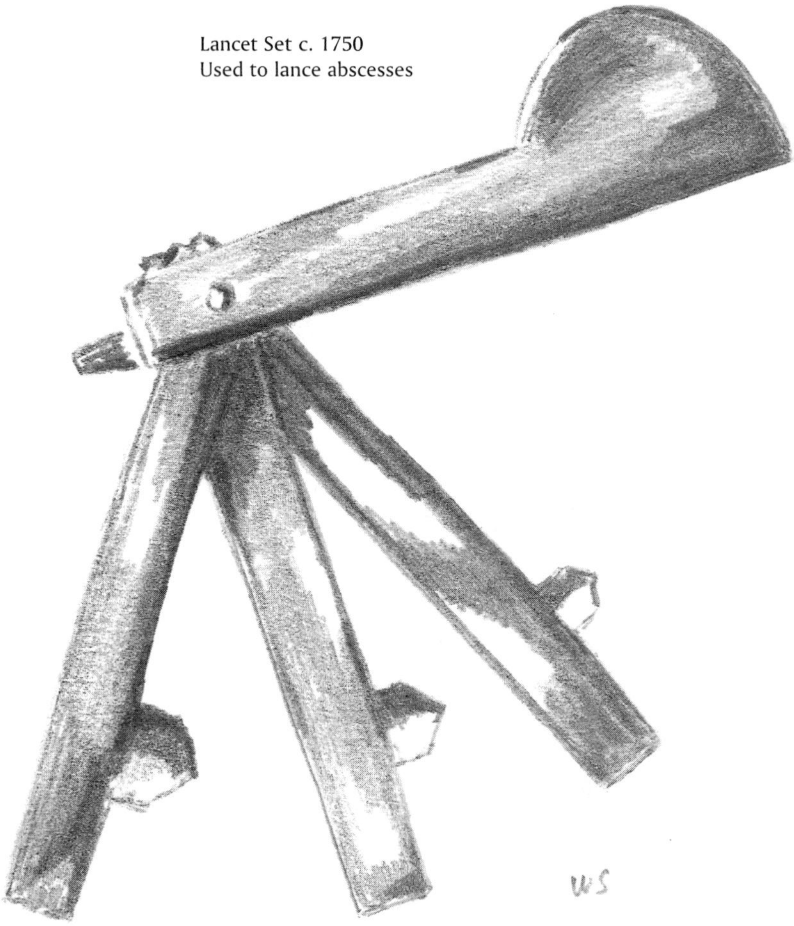

Lancet Set c. 1750
Used to lance abscesses

Chapter 3

St. Vincent Hospital

Green Bay was without a hospital in 1888. Operations and deliveries were done at home or in the offices of doctors. The acceptance of microbes as a cause of infection, availability of anesthesia, and the value of nursing were factors in developing centers of patient care. The medical and business community in Green Bay were aware of the need for a hospital.

The Businessmen's Association of Green Bay was actively involved in attempting to organize a hospital in the summer of 1888. One of the first meetings to organize a hospital took place in the home of Dr. Benjamin Brett. [1] A meeting of the Green Bay and Fort Howard Hospital Association met on October 26, 1888 and elected S. S. Murphy, president; F. Hurlbut, treasurer; and Dr. B. C. Brett, secretary. *The Green Bay Advocate* of July 26, 1888 noted the increased population, increase in manufacturing machinery-induced accidents, and the number of strangers in town as factors favoring a hospital in Green Bay. The August 9, 1888 edition reported that at least one business man was concerned that the Menominee River Hospital established at Marinette in 1883 had contracts with the lumber industry for patient care that took the employees to that city instead of Green Bay. Lumbermen could purchase a ticket from the hospital for ten dollars which entitled them to all medical care when sick or injured. They were required to pay an extra dollar a week if hospitalized. Marinette physicians also had a contract with the Peshtigo Company to provide workers medical care for one dollar and twenty-five cents a month for a family. [2] There was a concern that Green Bay was not providing adequate medical care for the community if medical services could only be supplied by out of town or by itinerant physicians.

Dr. Simon, a Kewaunee physician, was invited to the Businessmen's meeting of August 9, 1888 to give a proposal for a hospital. One Green Bay physician expressed his view that there were equally qualified doctors in Green Bay who were capable of organizing a hospital and there was no need to bring in an outsider. The proposal was rejected. [3]

Earlier in the summer, Bishop F. X. Katzer had been in contact with the Sisters of the Third Order of St. Francis in Springfield, Ill. He had suggested to the Businessmen's Association that the Sisters start a hospital in Green Bay. This suggestion, although well received, must have met some initial opposition because it was not until December before it was announced that four Sisters were opening a hospital in Green Bay. It would become St. Vincent Hospital.

The November 29 *Advocate* announced the opening of the hospital on December third, 1888. Sister Arnolpha Weber, Superior, Sister Wilhelma Broskamp, Sister Felice Hegemann, Sister Victoena, and Sister Eutichena agreed to care for patients of any religion and treat those who could not pay. In addition, they had to do nursing in private homes. These provisions were undoubtedly made to allay fears, expressed by the local organizers, that non-Catholics would be denied admission and infectious disease patients, if admitted, would affect others already in the hospital.

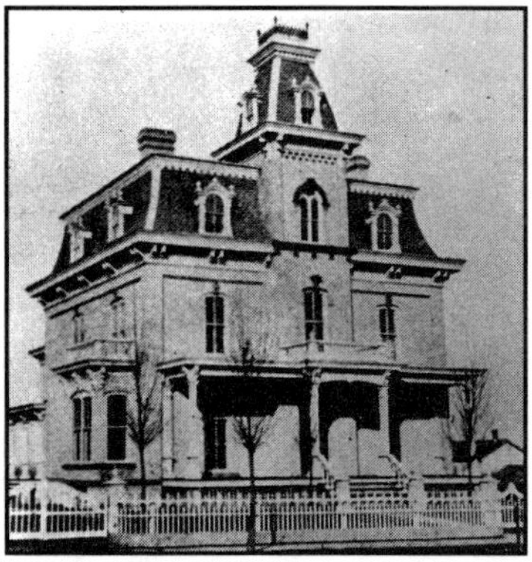

Photo courtesy of St. Vincent Hospital

The building chosen for the hospital was the former Dr. Van Norstrand home. Money for the purchase came from donations to the Businessmen's Association. The twenty-three room house of the doctor, who had gone into the lumber business , was located on Quincy Street. The house was sparsely furnished. One chair, four bedsteads, a rusted cookstove, and a big kettle for the laundry were all that was present. The sisters borrowed fifty dollars to buy a cow, poultry, and garden tools and started their mission to serve the sick. The home could only accommodate fifteen patients. The sisters did home nursing, usually for those with contagious disease who were not always welcome in the hospital, and for the added incentive to supplement their income. [4]

The first patient was admitted on December 15, 1888. Henry Kenny, age forty, was treated for kidney disease and discharged seventeen days later. Four other patients were admitted during the last two weeks of 1888. Diagnoses included sore foot, sore finger, spine disease, and cold. The youngest was age thirteen. The longest hospital stay was for twenty-four days. All recovered. Patient religion was noted in the log book. There were almost as many Protestant as Catholic patients admitted. [5] Total income recorded for the first fifteen days was $16.25, half in donations. Deficits during the initial start up were made up by monies received from the Sisters' base hospital, St. John's, in Springfield, Illinois and donations from the citizens of Green Bay. [6]

The following notice appeared in the January 31, 1889 *Green Bay Advocate*:

St. Vincent's Hospital, Green, Bay Wisconsin

Received of ________ Five Dollars, which entitles him upon presentation of this certificate, to admission, treatment, medicine and board in St. Vincent's Hospital, Green Bay, Wis at any time during one year from date hereof, in consequence of wound, injury, or sickness hereafter received or contracted, disabling him from manual labor, subject to conditions endorsed hereon and signed by him.

St. Vincent's Hospital

Sister Arnolpha, Superior

Countersigned ________ Agent

On the reverse side was printed:

Conditions. Insanity, chronic, contagious, infectious, and venereal diseases; also any injury existing before the date of this certificate, or arising from fighting or intoxication, are excluded from hospital benefits under this contract. This certificate is not transferable, and any person attempting to use it will be prosecuted. [7]

The tickets were a source of income to meet expenses not covered by patient payments although most of the admissions were not ticket holders. The ticket was good for all the hospitals served by the Sisters. St. Vincent also was the seamen's hospital. Sailors were frequently admitted, but their ability to pay may have been limited.

Only rarely did a patient die in the hospital. The first death was a twenty-four year old with erysipelas. Three others died within the next year. The diagnoses included broken leg, cancer, and tumor. Operations were still rarely done in the hospital until 1893. Broken bones and a rare amputation were listed in the log. Common diagnoses included respiratory infection, fever from various causes, rheumatism, and sore back or limb. [8]

Much of the care of the sick in the community was still done in the home. Confinement and births took place in the home. Most deaths occurred at home, also. There were many deaths of children and infants from infectious diseases including diphtheria and fevers of unknown origin. Often two or three children in the same household died from infectious disease within days of each other. Recovery from infection or accidents that could be related to surgery was noteworthy.

Dr. J. R. Minahan successfully removed an abscess from the lower leg of a boy in February 1893 at St. Vincent Hospital. A successful tracheotomy on a child with diphtheria was reported March 9, 1893. Dr. Ben C. Brett and Dr. Slaughter performed the procedure and the child recovered. The news article did not specify where the operation took place.

Despite the presence of St. Vincent Hospital, there was a perceived need for another hospital in Green Bay. Two additional attempts at hospitals were initiated in 1893-4. "Montrose Hospital" was started by two nurses, Miss Mame Wagner and Miss Julia Skidmore. The Henry Baker home on Main Street was configured for this purpose in 1893. Some of the first abdominal surgery was reportedly accomplished there. The hospital did not prosper and was closed. [9]

Dr. Slaughter and Dr. F. L. Lewis opened the Fox River Sanitarium Hospital on Shawano Avenue in Fort Howard in 1893. It was open to all physicians but for unknown reasons closed in 1894 and Dr. Lewis shortly left the city. Dr. Abbott William Slaughter had opened his office in 1891 and was associated with Dr. Lewis for less than two years. A graduate of St. Louis Medical School, Dr. Slaughter had practiced in Missouri for six years and then did further study at Louisville College of Physicians and Surgeons before settling in Green Bay. Dr. Slaughter was commended for his work during the smallpox epidemic of 1893. "He was chief attending physician upon patients who were then stricken, and his pains-taking attention to those in charge, also his prompt and wisely ordered and successful precautions to prevent the spread of the disease, won for him the unqualified praise of the people and press of the city, and was a praise richly merited." [10]

The *Green Bay Advocate* in the 1890s was filled with advertisements for potions and lotions that could cure a multitude of illnesses. A number of physicians from out of town held scheduled clinics at local hotels. Undoubtedly, they were able to capitalize on the high rate of incurable sickness with their claims.

Dr. Walter Lyman, a "magnetic physician" from Chicago advertised himself as a specialist in treatment of chronic diseases. He claimed to cure cancer without the knife, and epilepsy in a short time, guaranteed. He also treated diseases of women and men. The latter diseases included errors of youth that make them unfit for marriage. Dr. Turpin, also of Chicago, advertised as a surgeon for diseases of women and men. He would perform operations at the patient's home or at his private hospital in Chicago. He could positively cure cancer without pain or knife. [11]

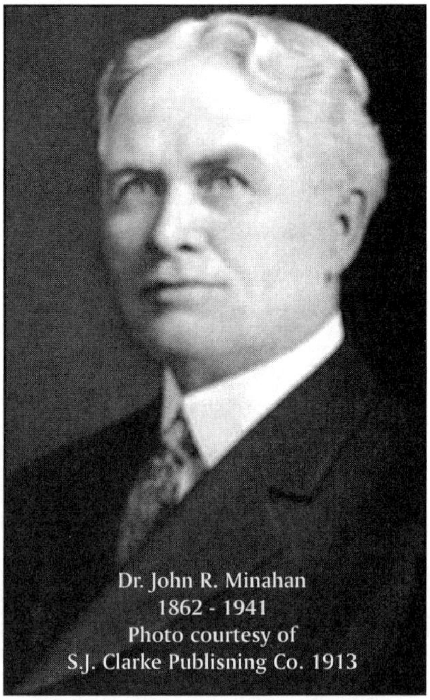

Dr. John R. Minahan
1862 - 1941
Photo courtesy of
S.J. Clarke Publisning Co. 1913

Dr. John R. Minahan arrived in Green Bay in 1891. Born in Calumet County of Irish immigrants, he was educated in the Chilton schools and attended the State Normal School at Oshkosh. He taught school in Mequon before entering and graduating from Rush Medical College in 1889. Classmates elected him president of his class. After receiving his MD he began practice in Casco before moving to Green Bay. He was 29 years old. It did not take long for Dr. Minahan to achieve local prominence as a surgeon. Six years later, in 1897, the following was written. "The doctor is one who, in his mere presence, is a tonic to his suffering patients. He is large of stature, of great physical vigor- a strong self-poised, self reliant personality who invites and compels confidence. He is a master in his profession, and this quality of belief in himself and in his own ability when confronted with a difficult case, proves an intangible, but none the less real benefit and help to every patient whom he treats." [12] Dr. John Minahan had rapidly established his presence in Green Bay.

Dr. J. R. Minahan also made a presentation to the State Medical society in 1894 on "Surgical Treatment of the Varix" (excision of varicose leg veins). Usually, a selected physician read a paper on a topic of interest to the members and then a panel of fellow physicians discussed the findings, giving their own experience on the subject. It was a means of receiving recognition and educating attendees. [13]

In 1893, Dr. William E. Fairfield, a native of Quebec, Canada began practice. He graduated from University of Bishops's College in 1886. The faculty of medicine bestowed two medals on Dr. Fairfield for achieving the best examination in surgery and highest score in all exams. Dr. Fairfield would become instrumental in founding St. Mary's Hospital. [14]

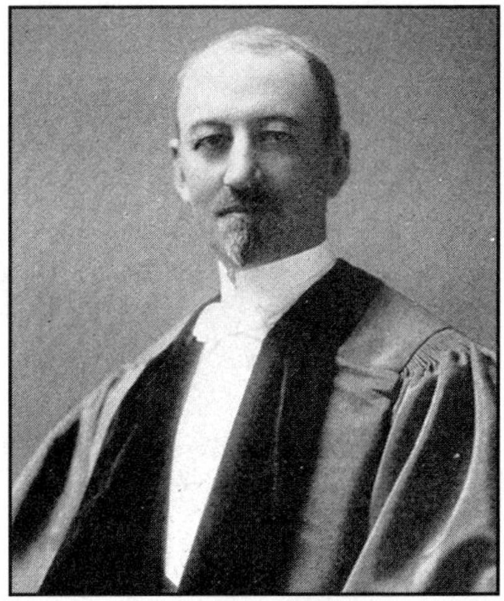

Dr. William E. Fairfield
1861 - 1942
Photo courtesy of
St. Mary's Hospital

The doctors who now entered practice in Brown County were better trained. Most had completed a regimented course of study in medicine at recognized centers of medical education. The preceptorship and reading of medicine trained physician was an entity of the past. More emphasis was placed on pathology, physiology and bacteriology. The science of medicine was beginning to be taught to medical students. Several attempts to establish medical schools were started in Wisconsin before 1900. Schools in Milwaukee for the study of medicine begun in 1851, and again in 1881, had failed for various reasons. Preparatory courses in medicine at University of Wisconsin, Madison were held as early as1886, but the MD degree was not awarded by the University until 1924. The Wisconsin College of Physicians and Surgeons established in 1893, became the Marquette Medical school in 1913. [15] Prior to 1900, most of the doctors arriving in Green Bay, fresh from training, if not European trained, were graduates of schools in Michigan, Illinois, or eastern medical schools. Few were Wisconsin trained. Brown County never attempted a medical training program leading to an MD degree.

The state of Wisconsin passed a law in 1878 to prevent non-diploma doctors from collecting fees. A doctor had to have a diploma from a Medical Society or College to be able to accept a fee from patients. This was an attempt to control the practice of unqualified practitioners. Not until three years later, did the legislature authorize fines and imprisonment for violation of the law. It was 1897 before a State Medical Board of Examiners and Licenses was formed. MD's, eclectic, homeopaths, and later osteopaths were included under the law. In 1871 there were fifty- two eclectic physicians practicing in Wisconsin. One hundred eighty-four homeopathic physicians were registered in 1874. By 1903, the State of Wisconsin had 2,500 physicians. Eighty percent were regular MDs, 14% homeopaths, 3.4% eclectic, and 2.0% osteopaths. [16] Green Bay, in general, mirrored the state-wide statistics.

Wright's Directory of Green Bay and Fort Howard of 1898 lists a number of new physicians including H. A Walter, R. C. Buchanon, Fred Edmunds, J. C. Kaiser, Albert Laing, Arthur Metcalf, William Nicholson, Francis Thibodo, and E. B. King. Very little is known about their education, years of service, or contributions to community. Dr. J. Doyle arrived about the same time. Dr. James F. Doyle was noted to be a 1886 graduate of the College of Physicians and Surgeons. For several years he practiced in Antigo, Wisconsin, where he also served as mayor for two terms. He left Antigo and received further training at Chicago Polyclinc Medical School, moving to Green Bay in 1895. For one year he served as an assistant to Dr. Minahan at St. Vincent Hospital and then started his own private practice. Dr. W. B. Coffeen arrived at Fort Howard in 1884 and moved to Green Bay in 1889. A graduate of Homeopathic Medical College of Chicago, Dr. Coffeen was described as "kind and of a sympathetic nature." [17] Dr. James Lenfesty settled in De Pere in 1897. A University of Michigan and Detroit College of Medicine graduate, he was remembered for his flair for staging 4th of July events. Eight oar crew races, polo contests, and auto races were apparently organized by Dr. Lenfesty at the July 4 celebrations.

By 1900, physicians were beginning to explore specialties of practice. Surgery, obstetrics, and medical doctors engaging in minor surgery only were emerging as separate practice models. There was no specialty training, however. Doctors would simply announce their own expertise and begin practice. Doctors were usually practicing alone or had shared offices. The hospital was beginning to replace the home as an operating site although home surgery or office surgery was still done.

Dr. W. T. Sarles lamented the passing of the medical practitioner of the past in his presidential address to the State Medical Society in 1900.

The successful medical practitioner of the past, endowed with a rich supply of intellect, judgment, tact, health, courage, and character, fought manfully the battles against disease, with weapons far inferior to our own, yet gained many victories and reaped the fruits of the conqueror. Though much of his fighting was in the dark, as ours so often is today, his qualities of manhood were prominent, and he was even greater than his profession, in eyes of the laity at least. He was respected and even revered, and his praises were sounded from one generation to another. He was family physician, not only to each person, but to the whole body of each member thereof. He was first to greet the newborn, whom he afterwards vaccinated, cared for through the diseases of childhood, followed to the war, amputated, trephined, examined as to his sanity, testified as to his ability to execute a will. and postmortemed; and even to the second and third generations of a family were his professional services sought with a zeal born of faith. [18]

Dr. Robert E. Minahan, brother of J. R., obtained a MD from Rush Medical School in 1886, practiced medicine in Calumet Harbor, Wisconsin for two years and then decided to return to law school. He received a law degree from the University of Michigan in 1894. Moving from Kewaunee to Green Bay in 1898, he began the practice of medicine and law in association with his brother. Six years after settling in Green Bay, Robert was elected mayor of the city. Robert served as mayor from 1904-1907. During his tenure, he achieved notoriety by ordering the city's illegal gambling devices to be assembled on city hall grounds. Before burning the machines, he personally destroyed them with an axe. Previous administrations had not been successful in eliminating the illegal gaming. [19]

Dr. Robert Minahan had an interesting hobby. He owned sixty-eight acres of woods three miles east of Luxemburg on which was he built a log home with a large stone fireplace and seven upstairs bedrooms for relatives and guests who helped make maple syrup. The Four Seasons Maple Syrup Camp operated under Dr. Minahan from 1910-1935. [20]

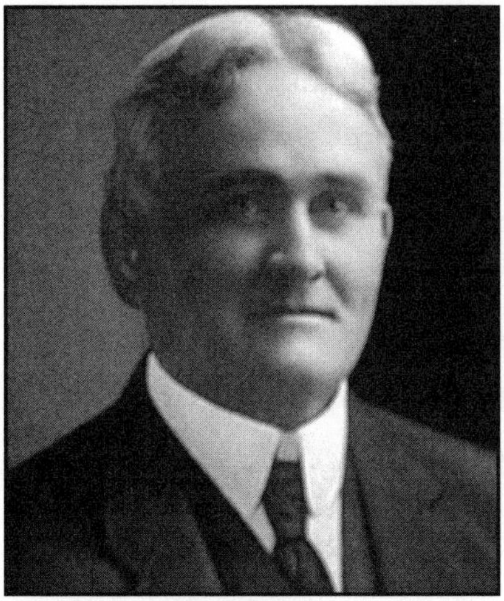

Dr. Robert E. Minahan
1858 - 1935
Photo courtesy of
History of Brown County, Past and Present
Vol. II., pg. 20
S.J. Clarke Publishing Co. 1913

The converted home that first served as St. Vincent Hospital soon became inadequate and the Sisters and physicians realized a new facility was needed. The number of patients admitted rapidly increased. In 1890, 116 patients received care at the hospital. By 1894 that number had risen to 410. The number of operations performed also dramatically increased. During the months of September and October 1894, sixty-nine patients were admitted and twenty-eight of them had an operative procedure. [21] The need for better facilities to accommodate the increase in surgery was evident.

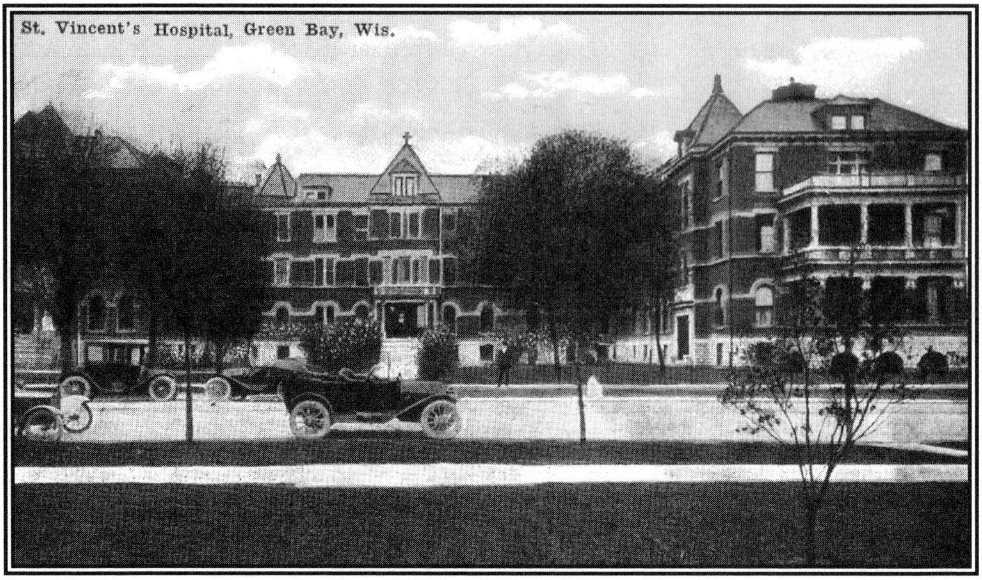

Photo courtesy of St. Vincent Hospital

The Sisters purchased property on the corner of Porlier and Webster Avenue for $3,200 in 1894. A new building at a cost of $27,000 was opened in 1896. Money for the project came from the purchase of the former hospital by Dr. J. R. Minahan and from the Sisters' Hospital in Springfield. Dr. Minahan gave the Sisters $6000 for the Van Norstrand home which included $2800 for the land on Webster Street. [22] The Minahans were generous contributors to the hospital in other ways. Their donations helped establish, equip, and staff their own operating rooms at St. Vincent. Whether other doctors were large donators to the hospital was not recorded. The large donation by Dr. Minahan probably helped determine the subsequent development of St. Mary's Hospital in Green Bay. Apparently, the Minahans were able to control who operated at St. Vincent and exclude other physicians from the operative suites for several years.

On October 10, 1900, five nuns from the Montreal Order of Misericorde came to Green Bay on the invitation of Green Bay Bishop Sebastion Messmer to operate a home for destitute infants and unwed mothers. The Order had successfully established this mission in Canada and were willing to establish a home in Green Bay. The nuns took over the abandoned St. Joseph's orphanage at 411 N. Webster and within the first year twenty-four women and thirty babies were admitted. Dr. D. J. O'Conner was the first chief physician and surgeon of the Mothers' and Infants' Home. Drs. W. Fairfield, W. H. Bartran, W. W. Kelly, William Nicholson, Fred N. Brett, and Austin F. Olmstead supported the Home during the first few first years. [23]

Dr. Kelly was born in Kingston, Jamica and went to school in Belgium before obtaining an MD from University Bishops College (McGill) in Montreal in 1903. Upon his arrival in Green Bay he was associated briefly with Dr. Fairfield. [24]

There were only two graduate nurses in Green Bay in 1902. A school of nursing was incorporated by the Misericorde nuns June 12, 1905, although lectures had started in 1902. The first graduation took place in 1906. Two of the first five graduates were nuns. The school trained three to five nurses a year for the first fourteen years except for 1917 when twelve nurses received their diplomas. The St. Mary's School provided a much needed source of nurses for Brown County. Hospital care for the sick and post surgical patients required more knowledge and skill than previously available from the most dedicated hospital matron. Dr. Fairfield assisted Mrs. Philomena Gryseels in writing a course of nursing instruction. Much of the teaching was done by physicians who were involved in the Mothers' and Infants' Home.

Dissatisfaction with surgical operating opportunities at St. Vincent Hospital probably influenced Dr. William Fairfield to ask the Misericorde Nuns to consider plans for a second hospital in Green Bay. Dr. W. W. Kelly also was instrumental in the effort to establish another hospital. The Sisters of Misericorde were not, at that time, involved in general hospital work but, caring for the sick was within the principal purpose of the Order. The Misericorde nuns also needed a source of income to support their Mothers' and Infants' home. Apparently, opposition to the hospital directed toward Montreal Bishop Paul Bruchesi came from sources "outside of the Order." [25] It is not clear where the opposition came from. Most physicians in Green Bay, excluding the Minahans, were in favor of another hospital to create more operating room availability. Reasons for the opposition may have been due to the fact that this would be the first general hospital managed by the Misericorde nuns; the nuns would have to solicit funds from the community and borrow money to build the hospital. This was difficult because the charitable work with unwed mothers was not fully accepted by the Brown County community. [26] In addition, the sisters of the Third Order of St. Francis may have been reluctant to endorse competition for St. Vincent Hospital. Dr. Kelly's father, Captain Patrick Kelly, a British Army Officer, and a friend of the Bishop of Montreal urged release of funds to build a hospital. In addition, Dr. Fairfield asked Sir William Hingston, professor of Surgery at Laval University, known to Dr. Fairfield from his work at the Women's Hospital in Montreal, to intercede with the Bishop on behalf of the proposed hospital.

The Sisters of Misericorde started construction of a new building adjacent to the original orphanage in June 1902. The two-story, sixty by eighty foot building had patient rooms on the first and second floor. The second floor had an operating room . The Sisters of Misericorde had obtained the permission of Green Bay's Bishop

Messmer but needed the Montreal Bishop's approval to release funds. Bishop Bruchesi finally gave his approval for the hospital on June 13, 1903.

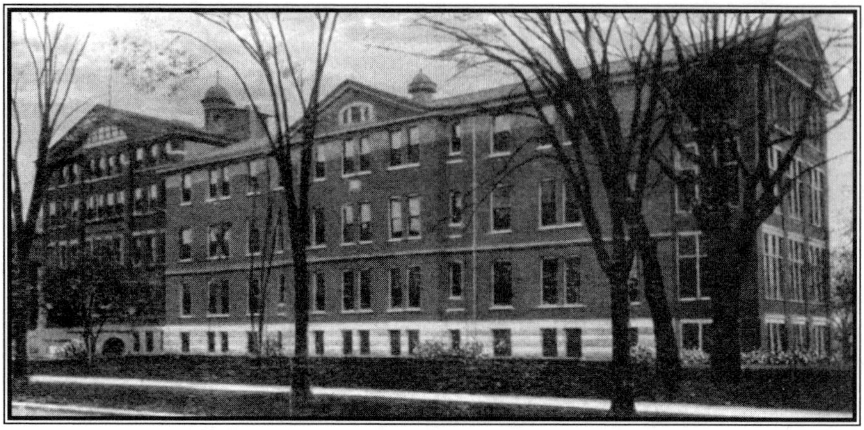

Photo courtesy of St. Mary's Medical Center

The result was Green Bay had two hospitals in 1903: St. Vincent located at 840 Webster Avenue and St. Mary's, three blocks away at 411 N. Webster Avenue.

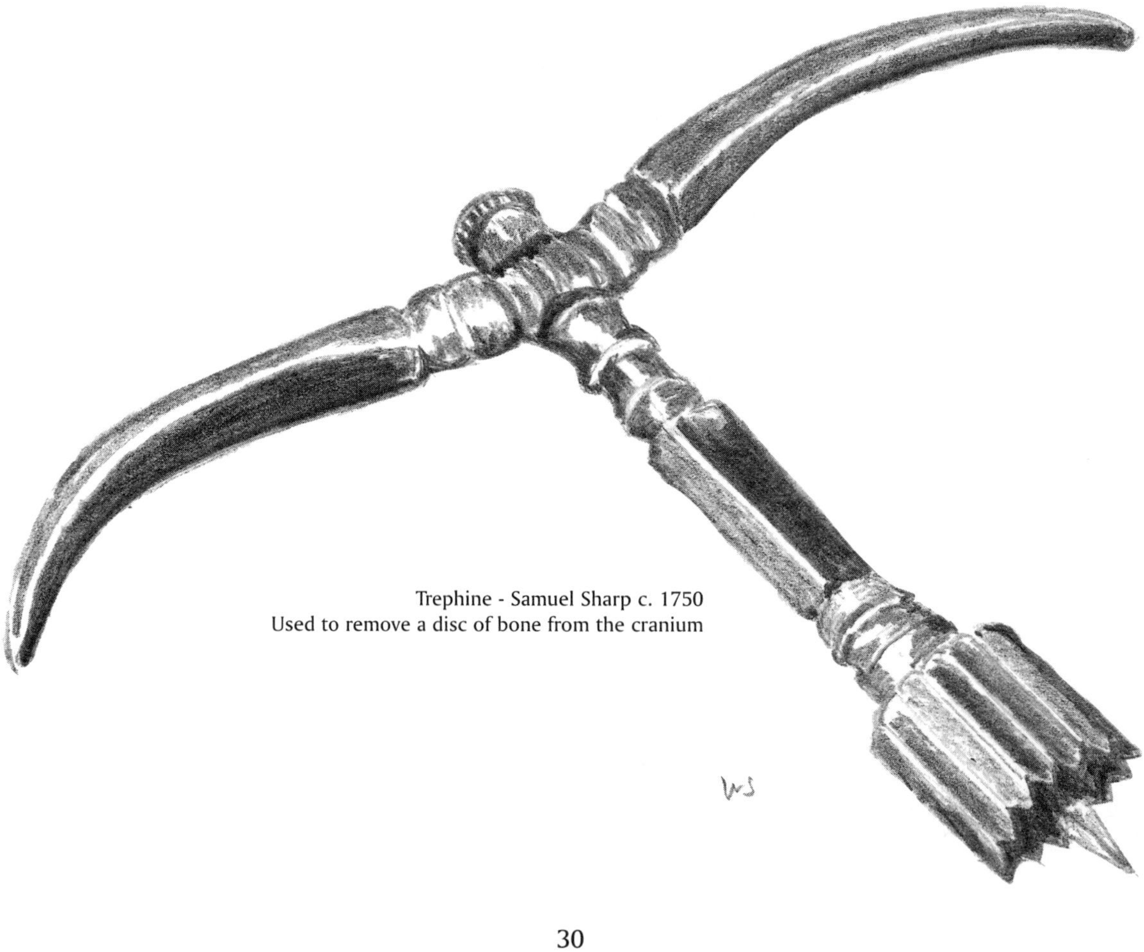

Trephine - Samuel Sharp c. 1750
Used to remove a disc of bone from the cranium

Notes to Chapter 3

1. Oliver, Dr. T. J., History of Medicine in Brown County, *Wisconsin Medical Journal* vol. 28, April 1929, pg. 159-65.
2 City of Marinette Centennial Program, 1987. Section on Medicine, pg. 31-34.
3. *Green Bay Advocate*, August 9, 1888.
4. Cook, Sister M. Francis Cook O. S. F. Ph.D., *His Love Heals, A History of the Hospitals of the Third Order of St. Francis*, Springfield, Ill 1875-1975, pg. 281-295.
5. Log of patient records, 1888-1894, Archives of the Sisters of the Third Order of St. Francis, Springfield, IL.
6. Monies Received and Paid Out, St. Vincent Hospital 1888-1894, Archives of The Sisters of the Third Order of St. Francis, Springfield, Ill.
7. *Green Bay Semi-Weekly Gazette*, May 27, 1902.
8. See note 5.
9. Oliver, Dr. T. J., History of Medicine in Brown County, *Wisconsin Medical Journal* vol. 28 April 1929 pg. 159-165.
10. *Men Who are Making Green Bay*, Gazette Publishing Company, 1897.
11. *Green Bay Advocate*, November 9 and 30, 1893. These are representative issues that had several advertisements with photos and positive descriptions of the cures awaiting the patient. Local physicians were limited to a business card with name, address, and hours.
12. See note 10.
13. Transactions of the State Medical Society, vol. 28, pg. 36-46, University of Wisconsin Medical Library, Madison, Wisconsin. Dr. Minahan was a participant at the annual meeting educational program.
14. See note 10.
15. Numbers, Ron and Leavitt, Judith, *Wisconsin Historical Perspectives*, 1981. University Wisconsin Press.
16. ibid.
17. *Commemorative Biographical Record of the Counties of Brown, Kewaunee, and Door, Wisconsin*, 1895, J.H. Beers and Co., Chicago, IL
18. *Transactions of the State Medical Society*, vol. 34,1900, University of Wisconsin Medical Library, Madison, Wisconsin.
19. See note 10.
20. Simonar, Carol, *History of Luxemburg*, pg. 127, 1983, Brown County Library.
21. See note 5.
22. Letter, Archives of the Sisters of the Third Order of St. Francis, Springfield, IL. The letter written was written February 2, 1895 to the director of St. John's Hospital who was overseeing all the hospitals under the Sisters of Third Order.
23. St. Mary's Hospital Papers, 1906-1953, Historical Collection, University Wisconsin Green Bay Library, Green Bay, Wisconsin.
24. Obituary, Dr. W. W. Kelly, August 4, 1951. *Green Bay Press-Gazette*.
25. *Green Bay Press-Gazette*, June 6, 1925.
26. Souvenir of Silver Jubilee of St. Mary's Mothers' and Infants' Home and St. Mary's Hospital, Green Bay, Wisconsin 1900-1925.

Chapter 4

The Appendectomy Cure

The number of physicians in Brown county was increasing and the need for improved communication among the doctors was recognized. Very few Brown County physicians belonged to the Fox River Valley Medical Association and even fewer had joined the State Medical Society.

The Brown County Medical Society was reorganized in February 1903. The constitution and by-laws were signed by Drs. B. C. Brett; Art Metcalf,; Arthur V. De Nevue; A. C. Mailer, De Pere; and Dan Gregory, De Pere. Dr. B. C. Brett was elected the first president. Other members who joined that first year were W. W. Kelly, A. O. Olmsted, Henry Rhode, Charles Stanton, John R. Minahan, R. E. Minahan , Walter Hagen, W. G. Nicholson, Abbott Slaughter, Mary Z. Vermeiren, W. H. Bartran, F. C. Brett, R. C. Buchanon , William E. Fairfield, H. A. Walter, James Lenfesty, Donald J. O'Conner, Charles J. Chloupek, Francis Thibado, H. M. Kersten, and W. H. Barbau. Members paid one dollar annual dues. At each meeting, papers were presented by members and discussed by two to three other physicians. Topics for discussion included appendicitis, rheumatism, carbuncles, ostemyelitis, and puerperal fever. [1]

Despite the addition of new members-Dr. Reginald Burdon, George E. Thompson, Richard H. Sweetman and I.M. Martin-only six physicians were present at the Brown County Medical society meeting of March 15, 1906. Those present discussed how to make the meetings more interesting and attract more members. Their conclusion was to read from journals and papers at the meetings. There was little encouragement for research or other educational endeavors. Further evidence of a lack of interest in academic medicine resulted in a resolution at a 1907 meeting of the medical society that deemed it unwise to develop a four-year medical school at Madison. [2]

The practice of medicine was changing. Diagnosis was becoming more important. The advent of laboratory procedures enhanced the ability of the physician to more accurately diagnose illnesses. In addition to very detailed observation and clinical signs, the analysis of urine and blood and body fluids gave the doctor a better understanding of the patient's disease. Fevers could now be related to a specific disease such as typhoid fever, malaria, tuberculosis meningitis, or tuberculosis of the lungs.

Despite the improved diagnostic acumen of the time, there were very few medicines available to the practitioner other than standard therapies of the past. Sir William Osier's *Practice of Medicine* published in 1892 suggested that pneumonia will run its course and is not affected by any known medicine. Treatment was mostly symptomatic relief of symptoms. Changes in diet, climate, and attitude were often all that was advised. Medication such as bromides for epilepsy, salicylates for inflammation, and mercury for syphilis were recommended. Curiously, Butler's *The Diagnosis of Internal Medicine* printed in 1904 does not discuss therapy. Fortunately, purging and bleeding, recommended in the mid-nineteenth century, was seldom used.

Preventive medicine had made progress. Diphtheria and tetanus antitoxin had been developed and smallpox vaccine was more routine. Lumbar puncture had been introduced as a method for diagnosing neurological disease. The sphygmomanometer, available after 1896, could measure blood pressure and X-ray would soon become a diagnostic tool in Green Bay.

Despite the advances in diagnosis and understanding of pathophysiology, surgery offered the only way to cure a variety of illness. Anesthesia was readily available and helped eliminate operative pain. Antiseptic technique, practiced in operating rooms specifically constructed for surgery, reduced post-operative infection. The abdomen could be opened and organs removed while the patient was under anesthesia. Better instruments were available for specific body area invasion by the surgeon. Nurses were trained to assist in pre- and post-operative care. Surgery now enjoyed more success in Green Bay because of the improved training of physicians and the presence of hospitals specifically designed to accommodate surgery. St. Vincent Hospital had enlarged and improved its facility in 1903 and in 1907 had added a new surgery department. In addition, St. Mary's Hospital had just opened a new operating suite in 1903.

The period between 1900 to 1910 was marked by an increase in surgical activity in Green Bay. With the opening of St. Mary's Hospital and a very active surgical schedule at St. Vincent's, patients from all over northeast Wisconsin came to the city for their medical problems and more specifically, for surgery. The railroads, also, influenced the flow of patients. Green Bay was a hub for major rail lines. Traveling from the surrounding communities was convenient. There was an influx of new doctors who began working at St. Mary's. Drs. R. H. Sweetman, J. T. Oliver, James Gibson, H. H. Hendrickson, Ralph Carter, and E. S. Schmidt, the latter a specialist in eye diseases, had begun practice. J. R. Minahan and his brother, Robert were joined by Dr. H. M. Hittner who assisted in surgery at St. Vincent.

Marie Vermeiren was the second woman physician to practice in Green Bay. The exact date of her arrival is not recorded although she did sign the fee schedule of the medical society in 1906. Her office was located at 319 Pine St. in 1910. She was still listed in the Green Bay directory in the 1930's. Her focus of practice was the problems associated with women's health.

A wide variety of operations were performed at the hospitals in the period 1900-1910. St. Mary's records indicate 2,821 admissions to the hospital during that period. Five hundred and six of the total 2,211 operations performed were for appendicitis. The next most common operation was currettement of the uterus, followed by circumcision, and tonsillectomy. Hysterectomy, both abdominal and vaginal, perineorrhaphy, ovaritomy, hernia, and abcess drainage were other common procedures. Gall bladder drainage was frequently done also. Unusual procedures included cleft palate surgery, hypospadias repair, nephropexy, pubiotomy, and talipes equinus correction. Cancer operations were more rare. Only thirty-three cases of cancer were noted among the total surgical number. Twenty breast cancers were treated surgically. The remaining cancers included tongue, cecum, cervix, and liver. [3]

Patients with medical diseases were less likely to be admitted for care. The most frequent non-surgical diagnosis at St. Mary's Hospital for the same ten year period, 1900-1910, was pneumonia, with forty-nine cases. Forty-one patients were admitted with a diagnosis of typhoid fever. Other infectious diseases, in lesser numbers, were admitted. Tuberculosis was the most prominent. Alcoholism accounted for thirty admissions. Rheumatism, nervousness, hysteria, neurasthenia, accounted for ten percent of the medical admissions. Surprisingly, there were only four cardiac diagnoses and an equal number of patients with diabetes during the entire ten years. [4]

St. Vincent's patient logbook from 1901-1905 shows similar patient profiles. The most common operation was appendectomy. For example, in November 1904 there were twenty appendectomies, three hernias, and three gall bladder operations. Of the eighty-seven patients admitted during the month, almost one quarter of the admissions were for appendectomy. Length of stay in the hospital was two to six weeks. Death was uncommon. There were two deaths during November 1904, one due to pneumonia, and the other typhoid fever. [5]

The Minahans had a slightly more diverse surgical experience at St. Vincent Hospital. Although gynecologic procedures were similar to those performed at St. Mary's, other operations including thyroidectomy for goiter and hyperthyroidism, prostate and bladder procedures, and tic douloureux were noted in the logbook. Deaths recorded at St. Vincent Hospital were also infrequent but did include what appear to be surgical cases and infectious disease. [6]

St. Mary's Mothers' and Infants' Home statistics from 1900-1910 showed an impressive maternal care record. Four hundred eighty of the total 483 births that occurred at the home during this period were delivered of primiparous mothers. "Not a single maternal death has occurred. This includes two cases of cesarean section, three cases of placenta previa, and other abnormal deliveries." Surgical cases were performed at the Home. These were cases requiring immediate care according to Dr. W. Webber Kelly, who succeeded Dr. O'Conner as Chief attending Physician and Surgeon of the Home. [7]

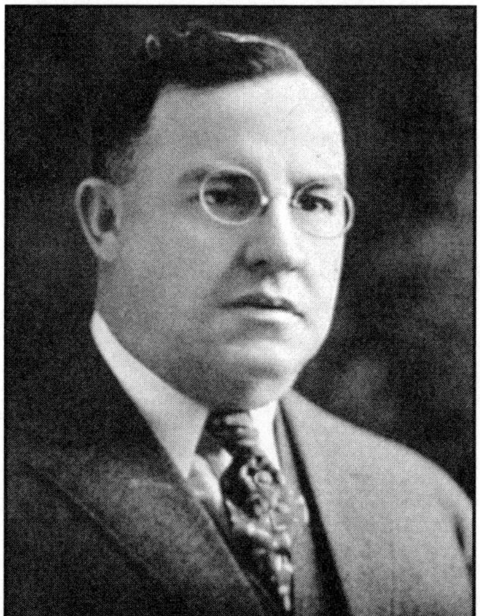
Dr. W. Webber Kelly
1875 - 1951
Photo courtesy of
St. Mary's Hospital Medical Center

The statistics for child mortality at the Mothers' and Infants' Home were not as good. Thirty- two percent of the 821 children admitted in the ten-year period October 1900 to October 1910, died. Of the fifty-three children that died in 1909, twelve were due to congenital syphilis, eleven pneumonia, and nine from gastroenteritis. The children born outside the home had the higher mortality. Many were in poor condition "due to days of exposure, weeks of incorrect feeding, and surroundings far from desirable." [8]

Dr. Kelly noted, "The infants entrusted to our care, entail an enormous amount of work and expense, and it is difficult to convince the general public of this, and yet when you stop to consider that we have as many as seventy-eight children at one time under our care, each calling for and receiving individual attention, with an average of twenty mothers or prospective mothers to be fed and clothed some idea can be obtained of our difficulties." [9] The Sisters of Misericorde received financial help from the community and were assisted in caring for the mothers and infants by nurses in training. Dr. Kelly, in his ten-year summary of the activity of the Home, expressed his sincere appreciation to the Sisters for their hard work and dedication.

Notes to Chapter Four

1. Brown County Medical Society minutes, 1903-1927. Hand written minutes of the initial society meetings are located in the Archives of the State Historical Society, Madison, Wisconsin.
2. ibid.
3. Ten Year Report of St. Mary's Mothers' and Infants' Home and Training School for Nurses, 1900-1910. Wisconsin Historical Society Pamphlet Collection, Madison, Wisconsin.
4. ibid.
5. Patient Log, St. Vincent Hospital, 1901-1904. Record of patients, diagnosis, length of stay, religion, and occupation. Also noted was whether the patient was operated on or died. The log does not identify the physician who admitted each patient.
6. ibid.
7. See note 3.
8. ibid.
9. ibid.

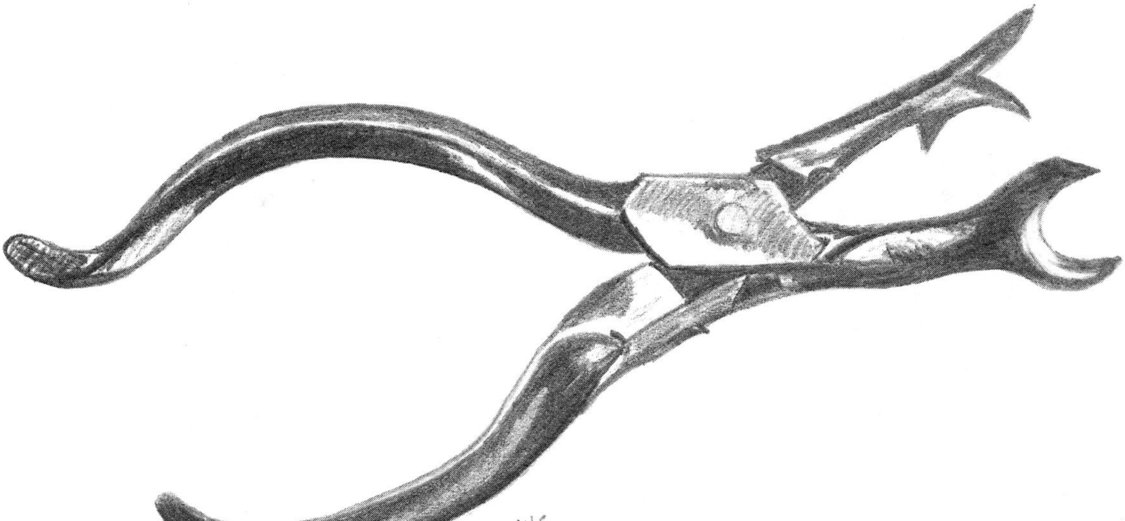

Forceps to remove trephined cranial bone c. 1750

Chapter 5

The Surgeons

The period 1900-1920 were the golden years of surgery in Green Bay. A surgeon could operate on a multitude of conditions using anesthesia in a clean operating room. His scalpel could cure appendicitis, gall stones, or a strangulated hernia. The State of Wisconsin required physician licensing but there were no restrictions on what an MD could do in the operating room. A physician, regardless of training or experience, could perform any procedure if he felt confident in his own skill. There were no pathologists or hospital staff committees to monitor the results. The surgeon did not have to keep detailed operative reports nor did the hospital have any means of verifying outcomes. Favorable reputations were quickly established by word of mouth. Patients as far north as Escanaba, south to Neenah, and west to Wausau, came to Green Bay for their medical problems. The patients were grateful and paid the doctor according to their means. There were no income taxes. The doctor could easily acquire wealth if he kept busy operating.

Two men emerged as successful surgeons. Dr. J. R. Minahan had already established himself as an excellent surgeon and businessman before the turn of the century. Operating at St. Vincent's Hospital, his reputation and hard work had built a large regional practice. Dr. Julius Bellin arrived in Green Bay in 1904. He quickly developed his own reputation for surgical and financial success. These two men would become rivals in an era of surgical eminence. Their entry into the medical field had many parallels. Both were progeny of European immigrants, were raised in rural Northeast, Wisconsin, and had taught school before entering medical school.

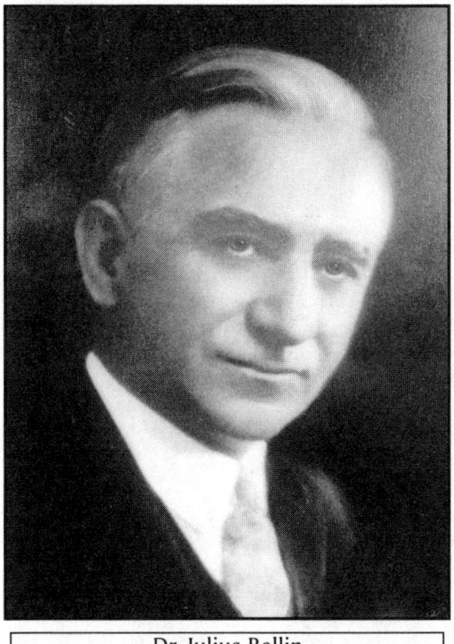

Dr. Julius Bellin
1870 - 1928
Photo courtesy of
Bellin Health

Julius Bellin was born in 1870 on a farm in Lincoln, Wisconsin. His father, Isadore, was a Belgian immigrant farmer and later, a store and saloon owner. Julius went to public school in Kewaunee until the eighth grade. Further education was obtained at Oshkosh Normal School and Northern Indiana Normal School. He then taught school to earn enough money to enter the Iowa State Medical College at Keokuk,

Iowa. On March 11, 1896, he graduated with degrees in both medicine and dentistry. He was twenty-six years of age. Dr. Bellin practiced medicine and dentistry in Greenleaf for two years, then moved to Wrightstown before deciding to relocate his practice to Green Bay in 1904. He abandoned his dental practice within a short time after moving to Green Bay.

The first Protestant hospital in Green Bay was established almost entirely by the efforts of Dr. Bellin. The first year in Green Bay, Dr. Bellin did most of his surgery at St. Mary's Hospital. In addition, he traveled as far as Door and Kewaunee Counties to do surgery. He would often do an operation on the kitchen table in the home of the patient. Not completely satisfied with the opportunities for surgery available at St. Mary's and being excluded from St. Vincent's, Dr. Bellin purchased the General Hospital located on 112 Adams Street in 1907, from Dr. Fred Brett. The fifteen bed General Hospital was quickly filled with patients. The first recorded operation, removal of a hydrocoele, was May 6, 1907. Of the first 100 patients admitted between May 7 and December 14, 1907, eighty were patients of Dr. Bellin. Nine other physicians were responsible for the other twenty. Appendectomy, gynecologic surgery, and infection were the most frequent diagnoses. Patient stays averaged two to three weeks for an appendectomy. [1]

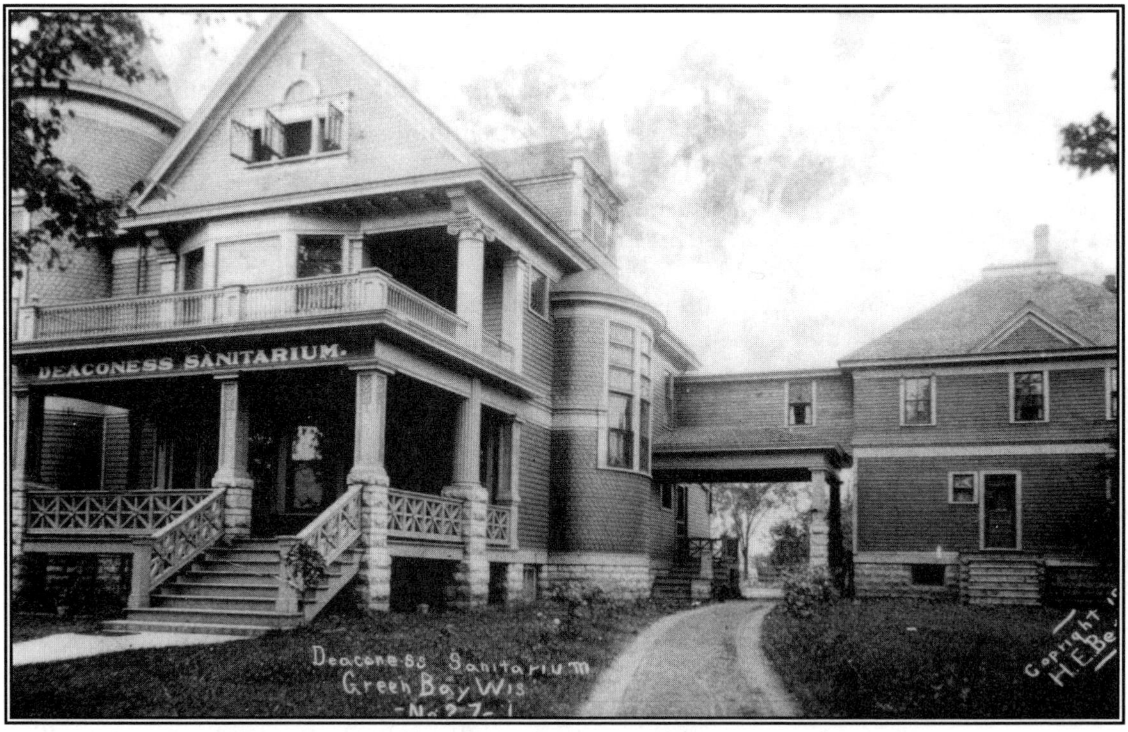

Photo courtesy of Bellin Health

Realizing the need for more help to run his hospital, Dr. Bellin contacted Mathilda (Tillie) Giese, a Green Bay native, and Delia Scheible, Deaconesses at Bethesda Hospital in Cincinnati, Ohio. They came from a Methodist-Lutheran background which sponsored the Deaconess nursing program. The two nurses agreed to take charge of the General Hospital, commencing on October 15, 1908. Miss Giese and Scheible were soon joined by two other Deaconesses, Hannah Wedewart and Carrie Krueger. From the beginning, it was apparent the General Hospital building was inadequate for the intended purpose. Within seven months, Dr. Bellin and the nurses were looking for better and larger facilities. [2]

The D. W. Britton home on Webster and Lawe was purchased for $10,000. Dr. Bellin spent $1,500 on remodeling the property for operating and hospital use. On July 1, 1909 the old General Hospital was abandoned and work transferred to the Webster Avenue site. The hospital was renamed the Deaconess Sanitarium and Training School for Nurses. The first nurse trainees were enrolled that same year.

Dr. Bellin soon realized his busy practice would require a larger facility and his search for funding led to the Methodist Episcopal Church. Dr. Bellin, who had been raised Catholic, joined the Methodist church to which his wife belonged. His position as a successful surgeon helped him become a very influential leader in the Green Bay Methodist church. Anticipating additional support for his hospital, Dr. Bellin approached the Wisconsin Conference of the Methodist Episcopal church, within a month after opening the Webster Ave. hospital site, to endorse the institution. They agreed. Before another year had passed, the General Deaconess Board authorized the facility. This meant that the Methodist Episcopal church assumed management and fiscal responsibility. The hospital and its annex accommodated thirty patients. From the beginning, the facility was too small, and discussion (presumably upon the recommendation of Dr. Bellin), by the lay hospital board was soon underway to plan for a new, more modern hospital. [3] "The present capacity of the hospital is only 30 beds. Double this number could be used. At least fifty patients have been actually turned away for lack of room this year, many more have been kept waiting, and of course, many more have turned to other hospitals. This ought not to be continued." [4]

The success of the hospital was almost entirely due to the hard work of one surgeon. Dr. Bellin was described as a "handsome, distinguished appearing man with eyes that commanded attention. He was charitable, friendly, and it was easy to work with him. Patients were attracted to him. He was dedicated to his work, had no outside interests, hobbies or diversions. He would work day and night, taking short naps between surgeries." [5] Initially, he did not bill patients. He felt if patients were satisfied with his service, they would pay and he did not charge patients if they had no money.

His associates prevailed upon Dr. Bellin to bill patients but he would discard many of the bills before they could be sent to his patients.

Dr. Bellin was very committed to his work. He was happiest operating. It was his life. Once he went away for a week and returned to find the halls of the hospital filled with patients waiting for him to operate. On another occasion, fearful of contracting syphilis from a patient on whom he had operated, he took an injection of Salvarsan (arsphenamine medication given to treat syphilis). Despite a debilitating reaction of liver inflammation and jaundice, he continued to operate, often while seated because of fatigue, during the two months of his recovery. He never did develop syphilis. [6]

His practice eventually outsurpassed Dr. J. R. Minahan's. It took over seven months for the first one hundred patients to be admitted to the General Hospital. Beginning January 1, 1910, only three months were needed to surpass one hundred admissions to the larger Deaconess Sanitarium. Of the first one hundred patients admitted in 1907 and 1910 respectively, Dr. Bellin admitted eighty in 1907, and seventy-one in 1910. [7] According to Dr. Bellin's own records, he treated and rendered surgical assistance to 1,067 patients in the hospital between August 1, 1918 and August 1, 1919. [8]

The competition between Dr. Minahan and Dr. Bellin extended into the business arena. Both men were respected and influential in the business community. Described as diplomatic, always smiling, even when angry, Dr. J. R. Minahan was energetically involved in many ventures. He was a director of Hoberg Paper Mills, Hudson Sharp Machine Company, Bank of Sturgeon Bay, and the Bank of Luxemburg. He also served as president and director of Peoples Trust and Savings Bank. During the depression, Dr. Minahan infused his own money into the Peoples Trust Bank to bolster investor confidence and prevent closure. At various times, Dr. J. R.Minahan was the surgeon for Green Bay and Western; Chicago and Northwestern; Chicago, Milwaukee, and St. Paul; and Green Bay, Sturgeon Bay, and Kewaunee Railroads. The position as railroad surgeon and the business associations assured a steady flow of patients.

The Sisters of the Third Order of St. Francis were recipients of the benevolence of the Minahan brothers. J.R. and R.E. were very generous in their financial support of St. Vincent. In 1907, the Minahans gave $1,000 for completion of a new chapel. This donation and other contributions were aptly noted by Rev. Zurbonsen in a 1926 article. "It is rather difficult to couch in words of praise and grateful acknowledgment the many services, kind actions, generous benevolence so unselfishly bestowed upon the hospital and its ministering Sisters by the members of the medical staff. It is greatly owing to them that the institution has attained such high standard of efficiency and great popularity. Will it be offensive to the modesty of the eminent surgeons, the Drs. Minahan who morally and financially have helped the hospital onward in its path of progress to say that the Sisters' community is especially thankful to them." [9] The Sisters did respond to the Minahan generosity by constructing a private surgery suite, dressing room , shower, and locker on the third floor of the hospital. A second floor surgery room with a dressing room on the first floor was maintained for the other surgeons. In 1915, a fourth floor surgery was opened and the second floor converted to an EENT suite. The Minahans continued to use the private third floor room.

Dr. Minahan's reputation as an excellent surgeon was enhanced by the railroad conductors. Patients coming to Green Bay for treatment sometimes were told by the conductor that they should be treated at St. Vincent Hospital by Dr. Minahan, the finest surgeon, instead of the physician they originally had contacted. Dr. Bellin on a least one occasion asked his associate to meet the train to be sure his patients were admitted to Dr. Bellin's service for surgery. [10] Rumor that the conductors were paid by Dr. Minahan persists to this day.

Another example of the competitive nature of practice occurred at St. Vincent Hospital. A doctor would admit a patient the evening before anticipated surgery, write the orders for the pre-operative medication, and schedule the surgery for the next morning. Upon entering the patient's hospital room the next morning, to his surprise, the admitting doctor would find the operation already completed, without consultation, by Dr. Minahan. When approached by the admitting physician, Dr. Minahan would congratulate the doctor for his diagnosis and leave the post operative care to the chagrined doctor. The doctor would not only lose the patient but the operating fee in addition.

St. Vincent Hospital census was growing rapidly. In 1894 a total of 413 patients were admitted of which 186 received a surgical procedure. By the year 1908, 1,808 patients were admitted and 1,067 patients were operated upon. [11] Although the surgeons are not identified, the assumption is that since other doctors were not allowed to operate at St. Vincent, the great majority of operations were performed by the Minahans.

Verification of the Minahans' dominance of the St. Vincent operating schedule is found in a letter written in 1950 by Dr. W. W. Kelly to the Mother Superior of St. Vincent Hospital. Reminiscing, he stated: "I was reminded that some forty years ago St. Vincent's Hospital was opened for the first time for general surgery among the practicing physicians and surgeons. Previous to that time Drs. J. R. Minahan and R. E. Minahan were the only ones who were permitted to operate in general surgery. All of our surgery prior to that time had to be done at St. Mary's Hospital which I was instrumental in converting into a general hospital in 1904. I saw the then Superior at St. Vincent's Hospital and explained to her that the Minahans would not live forever and suggested that permission be obtained from Springfield to open another surgical unit in the hospital for the other physicians. This was done, and the now present Specialists Department was finally built and equipped for the rest of us." Dr. Kelly was referring to additional operating rooms added in 1907. [12]

His reputation achieved, and a busy practice to maintain, Dr. J. R. Minahan was able to find the time and energy to build an office building at Walnut and Washington in 1907. At the time it was the tallest building in Green Bay. It housed medical and professional offices as well as a power plant for lighting. Dr. Bellin actually had his medical office in the Minahan building before constructing an office structure in association with Dr. Buchanon, across the street from the Minahan building. In 1915 the Bellin Buchanon building was constructed one story higher than the Minahan building. Eventually, Dr. Bellin bought out his partner. The building still stands on the corner of Adams and Walnut and retains the Bellin name. The Minahan building was later removed to make a parking lot for downtown.

There was at least one item that distinguished the two doctors. Dr. Bellin was vehemently opposed to alcohol consumption. This may have had its roots in observation of the patrons' behavior in his father's saloon. Dr. Minahan presumably did not endorse the same views as Dr. Bellin. An advertisement in the newspaper of April 1, 1918 made a satirical reference to Dr. Bellin's open opposition to consumption of alcohol. The ad was addressed to Mr. Julius Bellin. The last paragraph concludes:

Now dear Doctor, you say so many bad things about everyone in the saloon business. You are keeping the Green Bay Press-Gazette busy, telling people of Green Bay what an awful business the saloon business is. Now doctor, in fairness to yourself as a saloonkeepers son and in fairness to everybody in or out of the saloon business, would you be so kind and tell the Green Bay Press- Gazette how it really came to pass that you are such a good and noble man, a wonderful doctor but a son of a saloon keeper? I am sure that the saloon business did not make you a bad man because I know that you mean to do good, so please Vote for license as other fathers may want to educate their children out of the money they make in the saloon the same as your good father did for you.

Wishing you success, I am

Very truly yours,

J. J. Bins [13]

Both men had personal burdens to bear. Dr. Bellin married Lulu Vieux, a descendent of Charles De Langlade, mentioned previously as an early settler in Green Bay. Dr. and Mrs. Bellin's only son, Percival, contracted meningitis and was an invalid the remainder of his life. Percival was cared for in the home until his parents died. The residence at 637 S. Monroe served as office and home.

Dr. Minahan's first wife, whom he divorced, died in an asylum, his second wife, also divorced, was killed by a train while walking the tracks near her home. His third wife was his operating room nurse at St. Vincent Hospital. He had two sons by his second wife, both of whom died young. Dr. William E. Minahan, brother to John and Robert, tragically died with the sinking of the Titanic in 1912.

Despite widespread recognition in northeast Wisconsin, neither surgeon received lasting statewide recognition from their peers for their hard work and surgical expertise. In a 1976 article for the Wisconsin State Medical Journal noting the most influential surgeons of Wisconsin, these two men were not mentioned. Almost all those noted were from the southern part of the state. [14] Dr. Bellin and Dr. Minahan were active in the state medical society and were known to their peers.

Dr. Minahan was the recipient of extensive favorable local publicity for an operation done in 1923. A young girl had apparently swallowed a pin which had lodged in her chest cavity. During the operation to remove the foreign body, Dr. Minahan held the girl's beating heart in his hand. The girl recovered from the surgery. This was thought to be a first for a surgeon in the state. A detailed review of late nineteenth century surgery in Wisconsin by Dr. Joseph King suggested otherwise. In 1870 Dr. Solon Marks was credited with "suturing a heart wound" after removing a bullet from the chest. [15]

These were dedicated, conscientious, hard working men who dominated the course of medical practice in Green Bay and Brown County for more than three decades. Other physicians came to town during the golden years of surgery, but none could compete with these two surgeons whose legacy continues through the hospitals they endorsed with their surgical skill and financial success.

Notes to Chapter 5

1. Patient Logbook, Deaconess Sanitarium, 1907-1920, Bellin Memorial Hospital Archives.
2. Rudolph, Jack, Story of Bellin Hospital, *Green Bay Press-Gazette*, March 20, 1965.
3. Bellin, Julius, *Brief History of the Beginning of the Wisconsin Deaconess Hospital*, Green Bay, Wisconsin, 1919.
4. *Wisconsin Conference of the Methodist Episcopal Church Yearbook*, 1907, pg. 73.

5. Stiennon, Oscar, video tape interview with Dr. Lyle Edelblute, 1982, Bellin Memorial Hospital Archives.
6. ibid.
7. See note 1.
8. See note 3.
9. Zurbonsen, Rev. A., Institutions conducted by the Sisters of St. Francis, Springfield, IL., *Illinois Catholic Review*, 1926, pg. 78-80.
10. See note 5.
11. Hospital Statistics, St. Vincent Hospital, Green Bay, Wisconsin, Archives Third Order of St. Francis, Springfield, IL.
12. Kelly, W.W. Dr., Letter to Mother Superior St. Vincent Hospital, Green Bay, Wisconsin, January 27, 1950, Archives Sisters of the Third Order of St. Francis, Springfield, IL. Dr. Kelly was thanking the Sisters for hosting a dinner meeting of the entire medical community.
13. *Press-Gazette*, Advertisement paid ($33.60) and authorized by J.J. Bins, Green Bay, April 1, 1918.
14. Falk, Victor, *Wisconsin State Medical Journal*, vol. 75, April 1976, pg. 24-28.
15. King, Joseph M., MD, Historical Background of Wisconsin Surgery, *Wisconsin Medical Journal*, vol 56, November 1957, pg. 464-470.

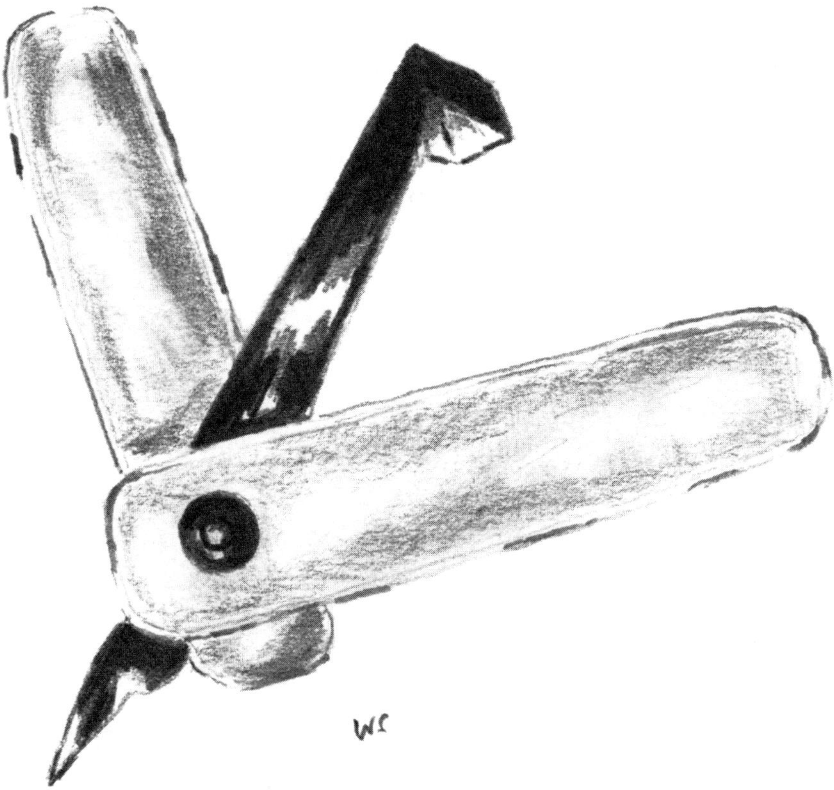

Blood letting instrument c. 1780

Chapter 6

Brown County Medical Society

The Brown County Medical Society became the unifying organization for physicians in the early 1900s. The three hospitals had separate ownership and to a varying degree each was dominated by a few physicians. Doctors had solo practices or shared offices. There were no hospital staffs or groups of doctors practicing as a unit. It was not unexpected that political and economic concerns would arise among the area practitioners. The only venue for discussion and action was the Brown County Medical Society. The Society expanded its influence later when Door and Kewaunee Counties were merged with Brown to become the Brown, Door, and Kewaunee Medical Society The county societies would not go their separate ways until the 1960s.

The Medical Society addressed a concern which potentially could affect their practices at a meeting in 1913. Members were aware of a contract being offered between the Moose Lodge and physicians in Green Bay. The contract paid the physician a predetermined fee for all medical services for a specified period of time. This was known as a per capita fee. Objections to this proposal were sufficient to pass a strongly worded warning to those who might be inclined to accept the contract. The resolution stated "No MD who does contract work for which he receives a per capita fee shall be admitted to membership to the Brown County Society. Any member (who does contract work) must resign. Members are not to aide he who was expelled." Soon thereafter, The Moose withdrew its proposal. [1]

Being a member of the Society was of economic importance to physicians. In 1909, Dr. William Wochos and his brother Dr. Frank Wochos who began their practice in Kewaunee, became members. For a brief time they had an office in Green Bay before returning to Kewaunee. D. Don Gosin, Dr. I. E. Levitas, and Dr. George Senn were accepted in 1910. Dr. T. J. Oliver, Dr. Reginald Burdon, Dr. William H. Bartran Jr., and Dr. Austin O. Olmsted became members about the same time. Dr. Ralph Carter, Dr. Robert L. Cowles, Dr. Emil Nadeau, and Dr. W. E. Leaper followed in 1916.

Dr. George Senn was a Green Bay native. His mother was a member of the Findeisen family. After graduating from the University of Wisconsin, where he received a "W" for playing on the football team, he obtained his medical degree from Rush Medical School in 1904. He continued his education and research, ultimately being awarded a masters degree in physiology from the University of Chicago. A unique accomplishment was a tie for the world record in the thirty-five yard dash which he held with two others. He allegedly was a firm believer in the value of exercise for his patients. He began his practice in De Pere but later moved to Green Bay. Dr. Senn joined the Army in 1917 and served in France as a surgeon at an evacuation hospital six kilometers from the front. At the end of the war, he declined an option to stay in the Army with a promotion but instead resumed medical studies at a French institution. Six months later he returned to Green Bay. [2]

Dr. A. O. Olmsted graduated from Hahneman Medical College in 1902 and practiced in association with his father. In addition to his medical practice, he served three years on the Green Bay school board. William H. Bartran Jr. was also the son of a physician. A graduate of Northwestern Medical School, he joined his father in practice concentrating on surgery. [3]

Dr. Thomas J. Oliver returned to his native Brown County in 1905. His early schooling was at the Fort Howard public school. He graduated from the Wisconsin College of Physicians and Surgeons in 1898. Jennie Brett, daughter of Dr. Benjamin Brett became his wife. Dr. Oliver published a short History of Medicine in Brown County in 1929. He also was involved in local politics serving as a member of the Brown County Board of supervisors for one year and four years as an alderman for the city. [4]

The Sisters of Misericorde appointed Dr. Robert Cowles to be in charge of the maternity hospital, day nursery and children at St. Mary's Hospital in 1919. Dr. Cowles was born in Wequiok, Town of Scott and received his MD from Northwestern Medical School. After an internship at Cook County Hospital, Chicago, he returned to Brown County to begin a practice focusing on obstetrics. His practice was soon interrupted by service as a Lieutenant in the Army Medical Corp in France in WWI. Returning to Green Bay after the war, he began an enduring relationship with St. Mary's Hospital.

Dr. Levitas was born in Marinette in 1885 and went to the University of Chicago and received his medical degree from Rush Medical college in 1908. A skilled surgeon, he was able to eventually emerge from the shadow of Minahan and Bellin.

The medical society passed a resolution in 1917 stating "the internal administration of alcoholic beverages be condemned as harmful in the treatment of disease." [5] Dr. Bellin, a firm believer in abstinence from alcohol, probably was much in favor of this resolution. Even under state and federal prohibition law, however, physicians were able to obtain alcohol for prescriptions and compounding medication.

Drs. A. J. McCarey, G. King, W. E. Mueller, F. L. Crikelair, joined the society in 1917 in time to see the annual medical society dues increase to two dollars per year. At one meeting, physicians were concerned that charity cases were not distributed equally among the doctors. The society wanted a revolving list of physicians to see charity cases to avoid over-burdening one physician.

Members of the society were urged to volunteer for the army reserve corps to improve preparedness during WWI. Drs. W. G. Fairfield, Don Gosin, G. King, A. J. McCarey, H.C. Mix, W. E. Mueller and George Senn were noted to have served as regular physicians in the Army. Dr. J. E. McGinness, and F. J. Gosin were in the Army but not members of the society. Dr. Eugene Knox and Dr. Frank Hager served in Europe during the war and came to Green Bay following the conflict.

Dr. Arthur J. McCarey was born in Antigo and graduated from University of Chicago and Rush Medical College in 1913 and then served a year of internship at St. Anthony de Padua Hospital, Chicago. Marriage to Arlene Joannes took place in 1914. He was in Green Bay only a short time before enlisting in the Army and being sent to France. A citation from General Pershing for "meritous and conspicuous service during Aisne-Marne drive of July 1918 when exposed to fire as Captain in ambulance service" and a purple heart was accompanied by a promotion to major. Dr. McCarey returned to Green Bay in 1919. [6] An active member of the Brown County Medical Society, he would become president of the State Medical Society in 1954.

Medical Society meetings were also a forum for discussion of clinical topics of interest to the members. Unusual cases and new developments in medical practice were highlighted in the discussions by the members or invited guest speakers. Topics included familiar diseases and new therapies. In 1922, Dr. J. J. Bellin gave a talk on tuberculosis of the kidney. Dr. Fairfield spoke on the use of insulin in the treatment of diabetes in 1923.

Another facet of Society activity was the setting of fees for the physicians practicing in Brown County and surrounding communities. These undoubtedly were general guidelines but peer pressure certainly would affect any extremes. In the April 29, 1919 Society minutes, a complex set of rules were approved. Hospital visits were two dollars, day visits two dollars, and night visits four dollars. The boundaries for the day and night visits were "North side; Green Bay and Western Railroad; South side, Chicago and Northwestern Railroad; East side, city limits; West side, Chicago, Milwaukee and St. Paul Railroad; and on Dousman, use your own judgment." Country visits were an additional one dollar per mile from the city visits. Office examinations were two dollars. Obstetrical fees were set at a minimum of twenty-five dollars which included all visits. Surgery for tonsils and adenoids were approved for twenty-five dollars. At a subsequent meeting in 1923, a charge of seventy-five dollars was the suggested fee for any laporaotomy. [7]

The Medical Society also attempted to set office hours and days off so that doctors could have more time for themselves. Office hours were to be limited to Monday, Wednesday, and Saturday evenings. Consideration was also given to altering afternoon hours to allow more time for golf.

The medical community did not always have uniformity of opinion on the issues facing the doctors. The normal competitiveness of medical practice could find resolution of conflict within the bounds of the society. At the February 24, 1921 meeting, Dr. J. R. Minahan broached the subject of closed hospital staffs. Many hospitals in the larger cities had a "closed physician staff" appointed by a select group of physicians or the administrative board and were not open to every qualified doctor. The ability of a physician to admit his patients to the hospital was more important than previous because home and office surgery was on the decline and the hospital could offer nursing care for illness not requiring surgery. Economically, hospital staff privileges were very important for the doctor. After a discussion involving Dr. Bellin and Dr. Minahan, it was resolved that the Society was opposed to closed staff hospitals. [8] Membership in the County and American Medical Societies, however, was a prerequisite to hospital staff privileges.

Notes to Chapter 6

1. Brown County Medical Society Minutes, 1903-1927. Archives State Historical Society, Madison, Wisconsin.
2. Martin, Deborah Beaumont, *History of Brown County, Past and Present*, S.J. Clark Co., Chicago, 1913.
3. ibid.
4. *History of Fox Valley, The Winnebago and Green Bay Region III*, 1930.
5. See note 1.
6. See note 4.
7. See note 1.

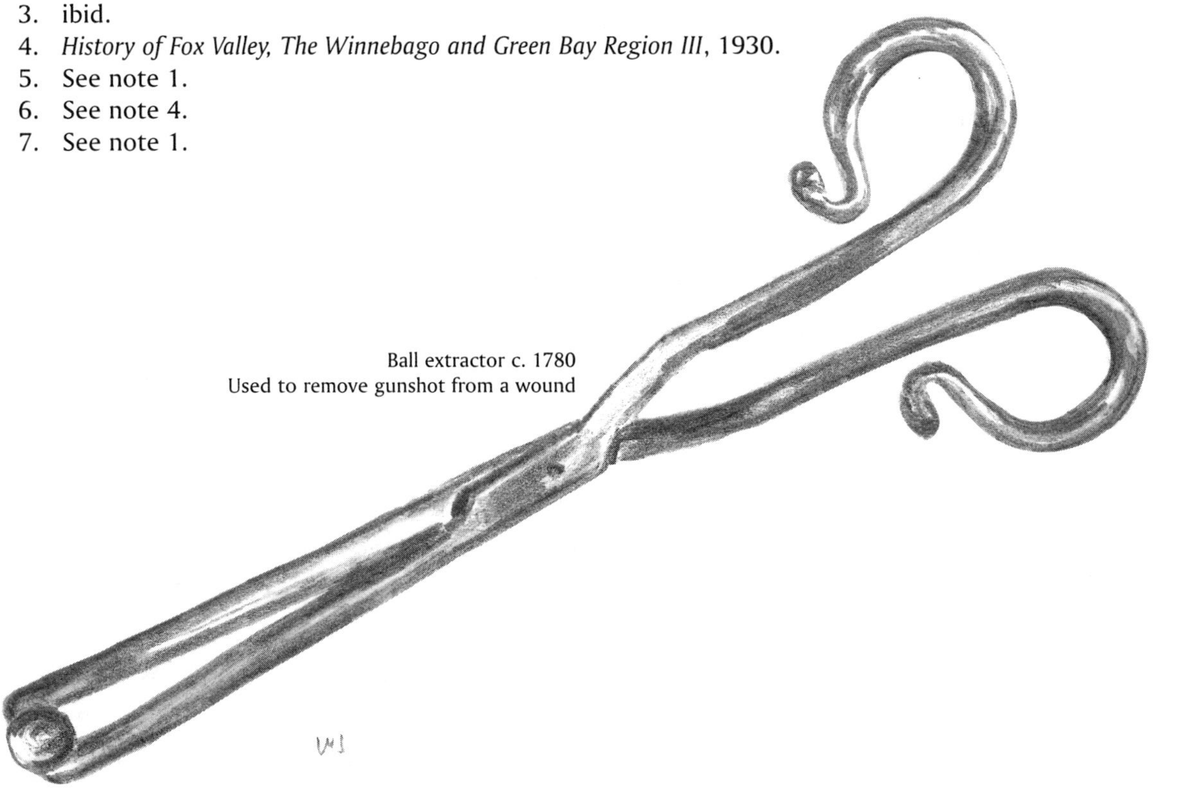

Ball extractor c. 1780
Used to remove gunshot from a wound

Chapter 7

St. Mary's Medical Staff

1918 marked the end of WWI and the onset of the influenza epidemic. Brown County was significantly affected by both. Returning physicians had gained experience in treating battlefield injuries and illness brought on by the conditions of the war. The lessons learned during the war were integrated into the civilian medical practice by returning doctors. This was the first war the United States troops had fewer deaths from battle casualties than mortality from disease. Nineteen of every thousand soldiers died from disease compared to fifty-three of every thousand who died from battle wounds. For every one killed seven were wounded. Early treatment of wounds, close to the front, was thought to improve survival. Careful antiseptic technique and organization of surgical teams were important factors in successful outcomes. Close attention to sanitation and prevention of disease helped lower the death toll from infectious problems. Statistics had improved from previous conflicts even though antibiotics would not be available to the medical corps for another twenty years. Influenza was a significant problem with the troops in Europe and at home. Military bases in the United States were particularly hard hit.

The influenza epidemic did not spare Brown County. The viral illness, labeled the "Spanish Flu" invaded Brown County in early October 1918. Four sailors from the Great Lakes Naval Band fell ill with influenza while on a trip with the band to Green Bay. Sister Loretta, a nun at St. Vincent Hospital who attended the sailors, died on October 4 from the very contagious and deadly flu. She was only twenty-three years of age. Dr. C. J. Chloupek, Green Bay health commissioner, issued orders the next day to close schools, theaters, Sunday schools, and meeting places. Health practitioners were ordered to wear masks in the hospitals. Dr. Chloupek claimed "one physician reported twenty-four cases of the disease in one day and the number of cases is one hundred twenty five according to the information I have received." [1] By October 23, twenty-eight deaths were attributed to the influenza epidemic.

Among the dead were two physicians. Dr. DeBoth, who also was called to see members of the naval band, succumbed to the disease. A graduate of East High School and Rush Medical College in 1911, he was thirty-two years of age. [2] Dr. William Krebs, also thirty-two, had been practicing in Green Bay only four months before being fatally infected with the influenza virus. A conservative estimate of the total cases in the months of October and November was close to five hundred sick. The number of dead directly related to influenza was approximately six percent of the total cases. [3] Fortunately, by early December the worst of the epidemic was over in Brown County.

The treatment advised was mostly symptomatic although aspirin, quinine, and Dover's powder (ipecac and opium) was suggested. Vicks Vapor rub was mentioned as a substance to rub on the chest. This was thought to bring the liquid formed in the lungs to the surface of the skin and relieve the congestion. A limited supply of a vaccine prepared at the Mayo Clinic was obtained by Dr. Buchanon. However, it was of questionable efficacy. The virus was particularly virulent and did not spare the young and healthy or the old and infirm. The residents of Green Bay were repeatedly advised not to panic. Dr. Chloupek reassured the public, " If men, or women, or children do not congregate in large numbers, the minimum number of new cases will develop and we should be able to eradicate the influenza in a comparatively short time." [4]

The enormity of the problem was of concern to physicians who were charged with trying to care for the patients. The influenza virus was obviously highly contagious. Isolation and strict measures to prevent the spread of disease were needed to protect the public. A "pest house" or isolation home had existed at 1701 West Mason Street near the outskirts of town since 1901. It was here that contagious disease patients could be isolated. The upstairs floor of the home was used to accommodate the ill. The first floor was the living quarters of the caregivers. Patients with smallpox, chicken pox, and diphtheria had been sent to the "pest house." Most were indigent and had lived in boarding houses. The isolation home was in existence until 1947. It served a total of 402 individuals during its existence. [5] The majority of the influenza patients were cared for in their own homes because the doctors believed better care could be given in the home. A few of the sickest were admitted to the hospitals; however, none of the hospitals were equipped to care for isolation cases.

Although Green Bay had an established health department, there was no full time person who could dedicate the time and effort needed to contain an outbreak identical to that which faced the city in 1918. Dr. W. W. Kelly, in a letter to the *Press-Gazette*, published in mid October, urged the city to consider a full time person to direct a fully staffed health department, a complete laboratory; and the building of an isolation unit as part of the existing hospitals. There followed a series of articles praising the suggestion but no immediate action was forthcoming as the epidemic was fading by late November.

The hospitals had been expanded before the War and had kept pace with the increase in patients. St. Vincent added a laundry and boiler house in 1913. A new wing was added in 1915 including a surgical suite on the upper floor. X-ray equipment and laboratory were housed in the basement. Deaconess Sanitarium was renamed

Deaconess Hospital and a new building completed in 1916. The new facility had sixty patient rooms and surgery facilities. In 1912, St. Mary's had built a south wing to the hospital and an additional floor to the original building. An operating room in the new addition was designated for the use of Dr. Fairfield and the training of the nursing students.

During the decade prior to WWI and for five years afterward there was a relatively rapid influx of young physicians to the area. Dr. Ralph M. Carter had established a reputation as a bone doctor. After graduating from Rush Medical college in 1908 and spending eighteen months as a house physician at Cook County Hospital, he began practice in Green Bay. He would become Brown County's first recognized "orthopedist." Dr. Arthur Charbonneau, born in Ispheming, Michigan, received his MD from Illinois College of Physicians and Surgeons and one year later, 1911, began his work in Green Bay. Dr. Emil Nadeau, born in Marinette, came to Green Bay in 1917 after a residency at the Illinois Charitable Eye and Ear Infirmary. He was responsible for starting the initial EENT hospital department in Green Bay. E. S. Schmidt, who began as a general practice doctor in Oshkosh and later received additional training in eye and ear diseases, was the first "EENT" doctor in town, having preceded Dr. Nadeau by several years. Joseph DeCock, a Green Bay native, graduated from Marquette Medical School in 1907 and began practice in Angelica before transferring to Green Bay in 1921. He served as the county physician from 1923 to approximately 1930. Dr. Frank Hager, a 1911 graduate of Marquette Medical College, practiced in Denmark. He spent a year in Europe during the War and then returned to practice in 1919. Eugene S. Knox spent seventeen months in Europe as a physician and returned to Green Bay in 1919. Born in Manitowoc County, he was also a Marquette Medical School graduate. Vernon J. Hittner, son of Dr. James Hittner joined his father in Seymour in 1923. He received his MD from Rush Medical College and had an extra year training at St. Josephs Hospital in Chicago. Dr. Joe Bellin, brother to Julius, spent a few years in Green Bay before leaving for the West Coast to practice. Others to come included Drs. W. C. Comee, Fabian Gosin, H. M. Kersten, Maynard Fuller, Louis Milson, and Patrick Minahan. There were thirty-five physicians listed in the 1920 Wisconsin Deaconess Annual Report.

Dr. Julius Bellin was president; Dr. R.C. Buchanon, vice president; and Dr. E. S. McNevins, secretary of the Wisconsin Deaconess Staff in 1920. Hospital charges were $10 per week for a general ward which included room, board, ordinary medicines, and hospital care.

1919 marked the first officially recognized hospital physician staff in Green Bay. Under the leadership of Drs. Fairfield and Kelly, St. Mary's Hospital was the first to form a hospital staff structure approved by the American College of Surgeons. This was an attempt to assure minimal standards for hospital care. The staff was to be restricted to competent and reputable physicians, not be involved in fee splitting, formulate by-laws, and hold monthly reviews of clinical cases. This involved a departmental organization with strict medical record keeping and review of operative pathology and autopsies. The hospital staff had more control over medical practices within the hospital and indirectly over the economics and scope of individual physician practice outside the hospital. Final accreditation approval was obtained in 1920 and St. Mary's became the first institution in Green Bay to achieve the "Class A Hospital" designation. The staff elected W.W. Kelly the first president.

1920
Medical Staff of St. Mary's Hospital
Green Bay, Wisconsin

Executive committee

President — Dr. W. W. Kelly
Vice President — Dr. H. Hendrickson

Secretary

Dr. R. L. Cowles   Dr. T. J. Oliver   Dr. I. E. Levitas

Surgical Service

Dr. George Senn   Dr. I. E. Levitas
Dr. R. S. Elliott   Dr. H. Hendrickson

Pathology and X Ray

Dr. I. E. Levitas   Dr. O. A. Stiennon   Dr. S. F. Rudolph

Internal Medicine

Dr. George Senn   Dr. F. Crikelair
Dr. J. P. Lenfesty   Dr. A. J. McCarey

Obstetrics

Dr. T. J. Oliver   Dr. R. L. Cowles

Pediatrics

Dr. R. L. Cowles   Dr. E. S. McNevins   Dr. E. S. Knox

Eye, Ear, Nose and Throat Department

Dr. E. G. Nadeau Dr. E. S. Schmidt [6]

"The past year has been a very vital one in the history of the institution, as it marks the inauguration of an entirely new system and the introduction of a complete change of policy in the management and conduct of the hospital," wrote Dr. Kelly in the Twentieth Annual Report of St. Mary's Hospital. He went on to say, "There has been a complete absence of that petty feeling of complaint and dissatisfaction which is so apt to occur in the introduction and running of such a system, and the present spirit which pervades the work is an assurance of still greater benefits to the patients and the scientific character of the work in the future." [7]

The hospital staff organization brought a new dimension to medical practice. Conferences and meetings to review clinical cases meant not only monitoring of physician activity but also the opportunity to review standard chart data for statistical purposes and education. Physicians were beginning to accept partial supervision of their individual patterns by peers.

St. Vincent's Hospital, including the Minahans, were opposed to the American College of Surgeons hospital staff proposals. The Minahans actually refused to talk to the representatives of the College when they visited the hospital. Reasons for the lack of interest remain unknown. St. Vincent would not develop an approved staff organization until 1954. [8]

There were other problems involving physician relationships which were indicative of the intense competitive nature of practice during the twenties. The Sister Superior of St. Vincent, in a letter of November 11, 1923 wrote the Director of St. John's Hospital in Springfield that Dr. W.W. Kelly wanted to practice at St. Vincent's Hospital and the Minahans threatened to leave if that occurred. Drs. Buchanon, Nadeau, and Bellin wanted him to practice at St. Vincent, but the majority of physicians reportedly were opposed. The sister reported Dr. Kelly even went to the Bishop to argue his case. The Sisters eventually informed Dr. Kelly that they would rather have him patronize St. Mary's Hospital. Apparently, the Minahan influence was strong enough to block Dr. Kelly from practicing at St. Vincent at the time. [9]

Dr. Bellin also was the subject of a different controversy. He was asked on January 4, 1924 to appear before the Brown County Medical Society "to explain any irregularities in his conduct in the practice of medicine." The subsequent minutes of the Brown County Medical Society do not record any further comments on the issue which presumably was satisfactorily resolved. [10]

Continuing medical education was addressed in Green Bay in 1924 through the formation of a new organization. The purpose of the Green Bay Academy of Medicine was to provide a forum for discussion of clinical papers written by members. Membership was by invitation only. A prospective member had to have practiced one year in Green Bay. His character, reputation, and education was investigated. If accepted, he had to present a thesis to be reviewed by the executive committee and defended in an open meeting. The first president of the Academy was Dr. A. J. McCarey. [11]

The 1925 fall program of the Green Bay Academy of Medicine listed the following: "Interpretation of Headache" by Dr. E. G. Nadeau; "Headaches Due to Focal Infection" by Dr. J. J. Robb; "Headaches of Nasal Origin" by Dr. Comee; "Optimistic Medicine-Preventive Medicine" by Dr. W. Wochos; "Gastric Disturbances Accompanying a Diseased Pancreas" by Dr. W. H. Bartran; and "The Relation of the Medical Practitioner to the Local Health Officer" by Dr. G. F. Goggins. [12] The program subjects were current topics of discussion and supplemental to whatever the medical society was presenting. The Green Bay Academy of Medicine noted its tenth year of existence in 1934 with a meeting on December 5. Presentations by Dr. Emil Nadeau on "Refractive Error"; "Pharyngeal Sinus Associated with Cervical Pott's Disease"; by Dr. W. J. Decker; and "Maxillary Sinusiti" by W. C. Comee highlighted the program. Unfortunately, this academic endeavor did not endure many more years.

Group practice was also new to the area. W.W.I had shown the organizational efficiency of surgical teams operating near the front. The Mayo brothers had started a group or clinic practice in Rochester, Minnesota. They originally had hired non-surgeons to help with their patient load but progressed to a group of doctors who shared facilities, patient records, and the expertise of specialists in surgery, medicine, X-ray, and laboratory. This concept of sharing extended into equal shares of the income generated by the entire group. The first group practice north of Milwaukee was formed in 1929 by Drs. Wendell Killins, internist, Carl Williamson, surgeon, Elverse Jordan, internist, Ralph Troup, radiologist, and within a few months of origin, Dr. W.J. Decker, EENT. Dr. Decker did not stay long and was replaced by Dr. Wilson Troup, also an ear, eye, nose, and throat physician. The clinic location moved from Main Street to above the C.A. Gross Clothing store on Adams Street in 1929. All of the members of the group were Mayo Clinic trained specialists. They chose Green Bay Clinic for their name and naturally modeled the organization after the Mayo Clinic. [13] The introduction to the Green Bay Clinic partnership agreement reflected the philosophy of the clinic model. "Whereas the practice of medicine in the past has been highly individualistic, but maximum efficiency in medicine, as in other lines of human endeavor, can not be attained by any one individual and success in the healing arts is dependent on the complete and thorough knowledge of medicine in the various branches; but the life span of man does not, in the ordinary course of events, allow the individual to acquire more than a small sum of the worthwhile available medical knowledge ... agree to form a clinical partnership ... believing it advantageous to form a group or clinic to promote the more efficient care of the sick." Each man in the partnership received an equal share of the profits. In addition, two weeks were allowed for clinical meetings. Rail transport plus ten dollars a day and the fees for meetings were included as benefits. A very restrictive clause prohibited a partner who left the clinic from practicing within one hundred miles of the clinic for five years. [14] These stipulations of the partnership would form a basis for subsequent partnerships of medical clinics to be established in Green Bay.

Most of Green Bay Clinic patients were admitted to Bellin Hospital. Although there was opposition toward a group of specialists practicing in Green Bay, the clinic was successful in establishing a large practice including many patients from the Upper Peninsula of Michigan. The financial records of the Green Bay Clinic from inception through 1937 reflect a number of economic realities of the times. The four original members of the partnership were able to double their salary within the first six months and by June 1930 were able to take in a fifth partner, Dr. Decker. The next few years saw a slowing of the Green Bay Clinic gross business but stability despite the economic depression. Collections were eighty percent of gross business in 1930-32 and rose to ninety-two percent by 1937 accompanied by a steady fifteen percent growth in business. [15] Apparently, clinic practice was accepted by the medical and patient community and most medical bills were being paid during even the worst period of the depression.

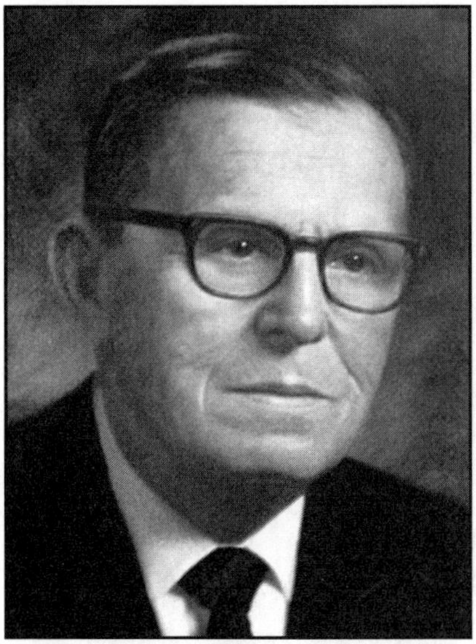

Dr. Ralph Troup
1896 - 1979
Photo courtesy of
Wendy Killins and the Green Bay Clinic

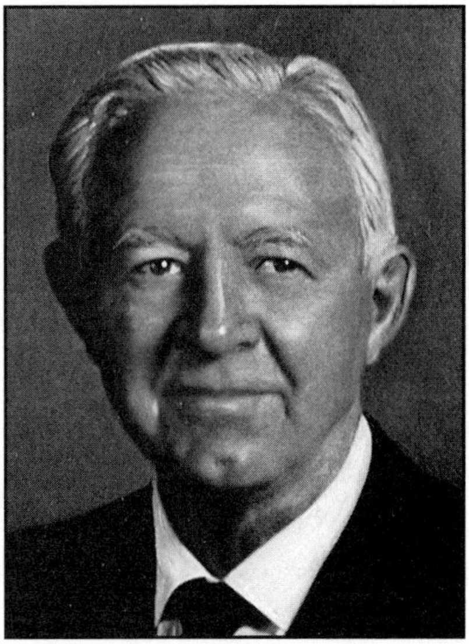

Dr. Wendell Killins
1897 - 1977
Photo courtesy of
Wendy Killins and the Green Bay Clinic

Another first for Green Bay was also instituted at St. Mary's Hospital. The hospital was officially designated for clinical training of doctors after they finished medical school. The American Medical Association had approved a one year internship pro-

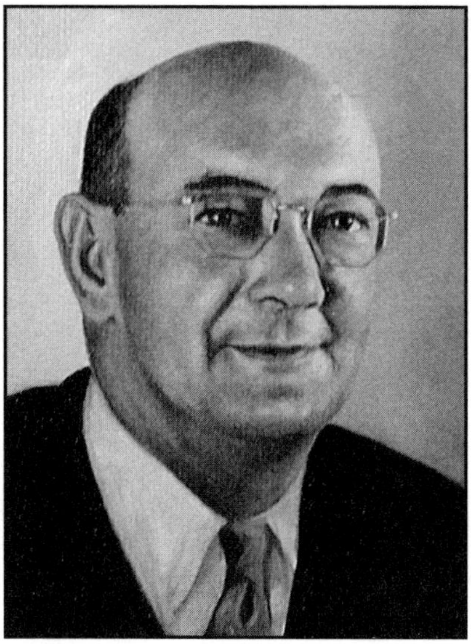

Dr. Carl Williamson
1896 - 1952
Photo courtesy of
Wendy Killins and the Green Bay Clinic

gram for the hospital in 1920. The first intern was accepted for training the same year. The internship program lasted a total of six years. Dr. Louis Milson was one of the last of the interns to take advantage of the opportunity. Of the six physicians definitely known to have been enrolled in the St. Mary's program, Dr. Milson was the only one who remained in Green Bay after completion of the internship.

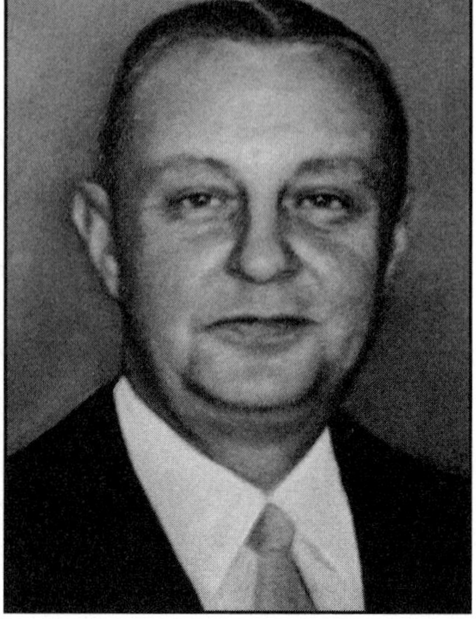

Dr. Elverse Jordan
1895 - 1955
Photo courtesy of
Wendy Killins and the Green Bay Clinic

"Persistence" was the word Dr. Louis Milson used to describe his pursuit of the MD degree. Born the first of eight children to a poor family located in the small Ukrainian village of Sokolow, Louis noted there was more "persistence" than food or clothing much of the time. At age sixteen he traveled to New York by himself to live with an aunt. He worked and attended night school to learn the language and qualify for college. Fulfilling a lifelong dream, persistence earned him an MD from Marquette Medical School after receiving a bachelor's degree from University of Missouri at Columbia. That same year, 1924, he became an intern at St. Mary's hospital in Green Bay. He apparently liked the city and opened an office on Washington Street the following year. His practice was slow to develop and he eagerly accepted night calls from established doctors in order to build a patient base. [16]

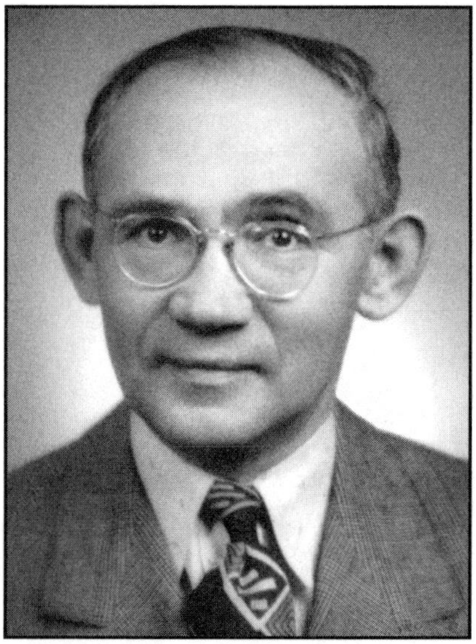

Dr. Louis Milson
1898 - 1989
Photo courtesy of
Bert Milson, MD

In 1926, Dr. Louis Milson and Dr. H. Hendrickson published a case report in the *Wisconsin Medical Journal* of the successful treatment of tetanus. The patient was a ten-year-old boy who had a puncture wound of the foot. The boy had developed two of the classic signs of severe tetanus infection, risus sardonicus and opisthotonus. Using intra-thecal and parenteral tetanus anti-toxin supplemented with morphine and chloral hydrate sedation their patient survived a usually fatal disease. [17] Dr. Milson also was the author of an article in the same journal on surgical treatment of obstructive jaundice. The case report documented the difficulty encountered when reoperating after initial gall bladder drainage was accomplished. Subsequent to drainage of a subhepatic abcess, the cystic duct could not be found and the patient eventually healed himself with a choledochal gastrotomy fistula, (bile drainage through the stomach). [18] Dr. Milson and Dr. Donel Sullivan formed an association that was in later years became the Dousman Clinic located near St. Mary's Hospital on the West side. Dr. Milson's two sons also became physicians, joining him in the 1960's.

Dr. Patrick Minahan (cousin) became an associate of J. R. Minahan and R. E. Minahan in 1921. Immediately after graduating from Rush Medical School, Dr. Patrick Minahan took over a rural practice for a short time while the doctor took a much needed vacation. The very first patient he was asked to see was a teen-age boy who had an abcess of his foot. After carefully washing the foot and sterilizing his knife with carbolic acid, he incised and drained the abcess. Calomel pills, to be given one at a time over several hours, were prescribed for the boy's constipation. Dr. Minahan left the farm house with the secure feeling he had done the appropriate therapy and returned leisurely to the office by horseback. In his judgment the boy would recover from the treatment. To his surprise, the father approached rapidly on his horse, crying his son had died and for the doctor to return quickly. Dr. Minahan, not understanding the reason for the unexpected death, returned and carefully reviewed the care with the grieving parents. The father already had questioned the pills as the cause of his son's death. He had given the chickens some of the Calomel but they had not died and therefor dismissed the medication as a cause.

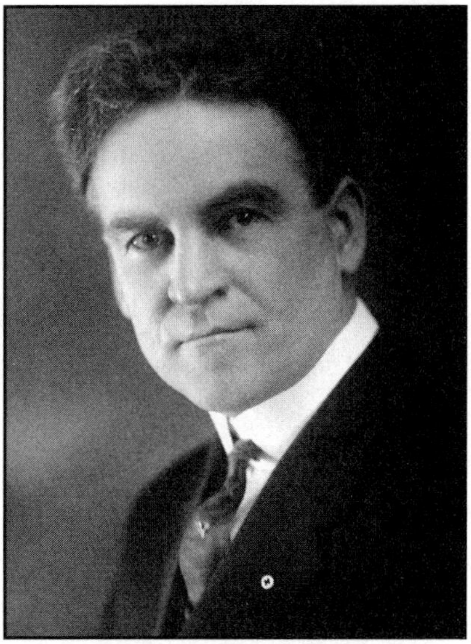

Dr. Patrick Minahan
1875 - 1953
Photo courtesy of
Wisconsin Historical Society WHi 4478

Dr. Minahan asked the mother if she had followed the directions for giving the pills to her son. Her reply indicated she had given the medication exactly as he prescribed. Then he asked her what she used to wash down the pills. Unfortunately, she had given her son the glass containing the carbolic acid which was conveniently nearby. The mother had unintentionally poisoned her own son. [19] Despite this unfortunate tragedy, Dr. Minahan was to become a respected physician and eventually president of the State Medical Society.

Dr. Patrick Minahan began practice in Casco in 1898 and moved to Algoma in 1905. Dr. Minahan left Algoma for reasons of health. He spent two years recuperating in Prentice, Wisconsin where he was involved in politics and the lumber business before returning to medicine. In 1912 he took over the practice of William E. Minahan in Fond Du Lac. After his military service in W.W.I he returned to Fond Du Lac. In 1921 he decided to join his cousins J. R. and R. E. Minahan in Green Bay. The association lasted three years before he established his own office.

Deaconess Hospital and the Training School for Nurses was continuing to benefit from the industry of Dr. Julius Bellin. In 1925, Charlotte Fowler, a graduate of the nursing program, donated money for a nurses' dormitory in the north wing of the hospital. About the same time, Dr. Bellin and his wife donated $50,000 to the hospital for a new four-story wing which was opened in 1927. The new building could accommodate one hundred patients. Recognizing his invaluable contribution, the hospital board honored the doctor by renaming the institution Bellin Memorial Hospital. At the time he was president of the hospital board. The Wisconsin Conference of the Methodist Episcopal Church approved the name change in 1926. Dr. Bellin was named president of Board of Hospitals and Homes of the Wisconsin Conference the same year. [20] Unfortunately, high blood pressure and heart failure would soon end the dedicated life of the man who was identified with the hospital bearing his name. Dr. Bellin was said to always have another project formulated before the last was completed. His goal was to build a crippled children's hospital and medical building in association with Bellin Hospital. It was rumored that he would donate another $50,000 to initiate the project. However, it would not happen. Dr. Bellin died September 26, 1928. [21] His will provided annuities for his wife, mother, and son. After their deaths the income from his office building was to go to the hospital as long as it remained Bellin Memorial Hospital. The real estate was not to be sold until 50 years after his death and the proceeds were to go to the hospital. His will also contained the wish that the hospital operate under an open staff of physicians and surgeons. [22] The legacy of Dr. Bellin continues as Bellin Health today.

Notes to Chapter 7

1. *Green Bay Press-Gazette*, October 5, 1918.
2. ibid, October 7, 1918.
3. ibid, October 23,1918.
4. See note 1. Articles appeared almost daily during the month of October, 1918 with updated reports of illness, deaths, and suggestions for prevention and care of the ill.
5. *Green Bay Press-Gazette*, August 7, 1948.
6. Twentieth Annual Report of St. Mary's Hospital and Training School for Nurses and of St. Mary's Mothers' and Infants' Home for the year ending Sept. 30, 1920. Archives of the Sisters of Misericorde, Montreal, Canada.
7. ibid.
8. Letter to Father Director of St. John's Hospital, Springfield, Illinois from Sister Superior, St. Vincent Hospital, Green Bay, Wisconsin, February 1, 1922. Archives Sisters of the Third Order of St. Francis, Springfield, IL.
9. Letter from Sister Superior to the Director of St. John's Hospital Springfield, Ill. who was responsible for the administration of all the Hospitals under the Third Order of St. Francis, Archives of the Third Order, Springfield, IL.
10. Minutes of the Brown County Medical Society, Jan. 4, 1924. Archives Wisconsin State Historical Society, Madison, Wisconsin
11. Green Bay Academy of Medicine, Constitution and By-Laws, 1924, Program 1924-1925. State Historical Society, Madison, Wisconsin.
12. ibid.
13. Killins, Dr. Jack., personal communication.
14. Green Bay Clinic Partnership Agreement Jan 1, 1930. Financial Records Green Bay Clinic, 1929-37, Archives, University of Wisconsin Green Bay Library, Green Bay, Wisconsin.
15. ibid.
16. Milson, Louis Dr., *The Story of My Life*, unpublished written about 1980, Archives Neville Public Museum, Green Bay, Wisconsin.
17. Milson, Louis Dr., Hendrickson, H. Dr., Tetanus Case Report, *Wisconsin Medical Journal*, vol. 25 1926, pg. 345-6.
18. Milson, Louis Dr., Common Duct Obstruction, Case Report, *Wisconsin Medical Journal*, vol. 33 1934, pg. 817-21.
19. Minahan, Patrick MD. 1875-1953, *Milestones of Memory*, Autobiography 1953, unpublished, Brown County Library Historical Collection, Green Bay, Wisconsin
20. Wisconsin Conference of Methodist Episcopal Church, Report of the Board of Hospitals and Homes, 1926, pg. 491.
21. *Green Bay Press-Gazette*, September 27, 1928, Obituary Dr. Julius Bellin.
22. Last Will and Testament of Julius Bellin, Brown County Library Historical Collection, Green Bay, Wisconsin.

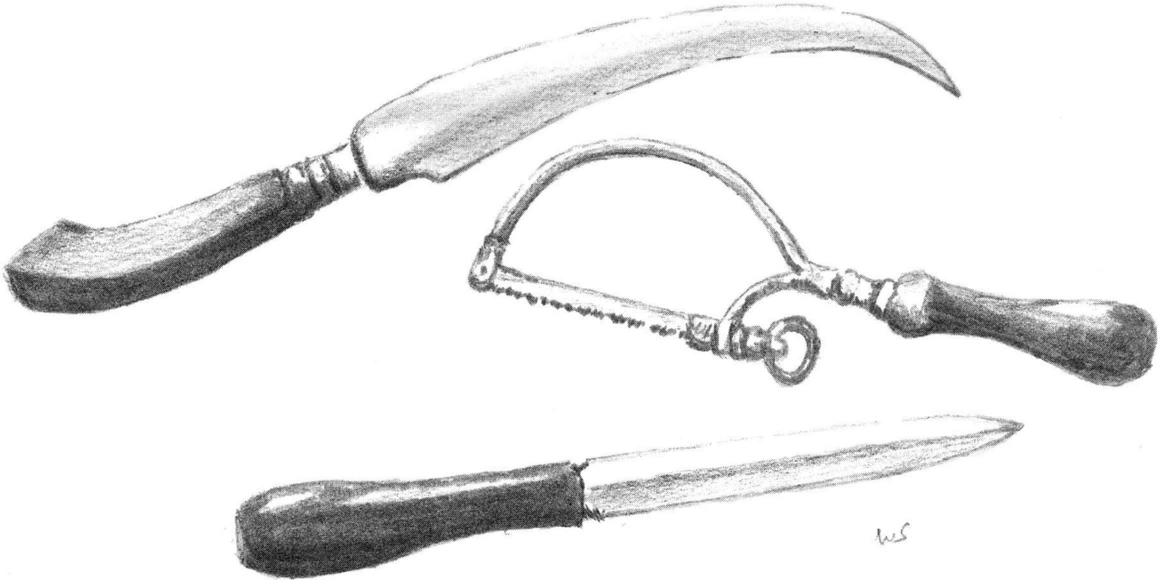

Surgical amputation instruments c. 1780

Chapter 8

End of An Era

Economic pressures and the Depression had a significant effect upon the expansion and modernization of the three Green Bay hospitals. A period of twenty years would pass during which time only St. Vincent Hospital would make major improvements in facilities. A building project on the northwest corner of St. Vincent Hospital completed in 1927 included Sister's quarters, private rooms, and dining halls. Laundry, boiler room, kitchens, and elevator were also installed during the period of 1927-30. St. Vincent's replaced the worn wooden floors with the hospital's distinctive terrazzo floors in 1930. An addition to the southeast corner in 1931 housed a new X-ray department, pharmacy and doctors' room in the basement, patient rooms on the second and third floors, and maternity department on the third floor. Renovation of the radiology department to accommodate an in-house radiologist was accomplished in 1937. The radiology department was equipped with new diagnostic X-ray equipment and an electrocardiograph machine was purchased for the laboratory. A 220,00 volt therapeutic X-ray machine was also purchased for treating skin and blood diseases. [1]

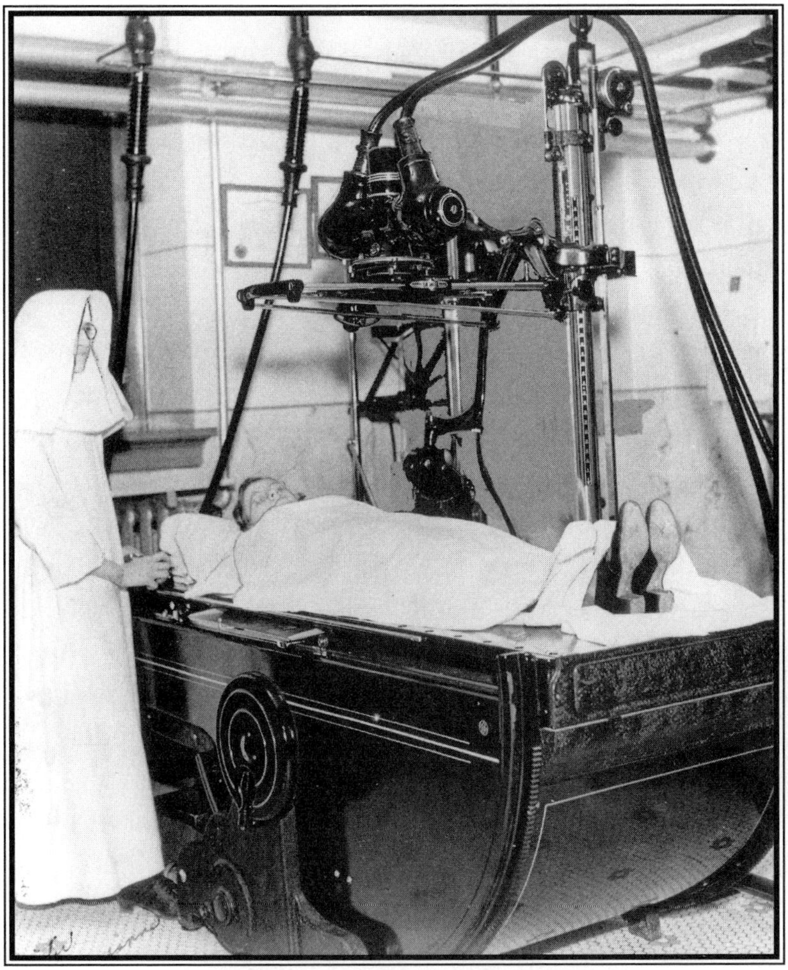

Photo courtesy of St. Vincent Hospital

Neither St. Mary's nor Bellin Hospital made any significant alteration in their facilities until after

WWII. A few new physicians came to town during the Depression and prior to the war, but the economy and war deterred construction of new facilities and expansion.

In 1933, Dr. J. R. Minahan apparently successfully opposed having a radiologist in St. Vincent Hospital even though the younger staff were much in favor. (The first radiologist at St. Vincent did not arrive until four years later.) At the time, the Sister Superior expressed concern that the younger doctors would hesitate to bring their patients to the hospital if a radiologist was not present to interpret films. X-rays were interpreted by the ordering physician or a radiologist in practice in the community. [2]

Dr. Oscar Stiennon expressed his opinion concerning the changes confronting the practicing physician in an article in the *Wisconsin Medical Journal* printed in 1934. He noted the individual physician's autonomy was being threatened by large organizations and government. The American College of Surgeons were criticized for standardizing training, hospitals, and nursing and promoting specialists. Group practice, "organized on a share basis, with a credit manager and other accouterments of big business" was denounced as lacking a humanitarian objective. The physician's prerogative to provide private charity to his patient, treat his patient with sentiment, and charge fees appropriate to the patient's means was threatened according to Dr. Stiennon. [3] Despite the success of the Green Bay Clinic, two decades would pass before the formation of other major clinics in Brown County. St. Mary's Hospital was the only hospital with an American College of Surgeons approved physician staff. This was still the era of fiercely independent family doctors.

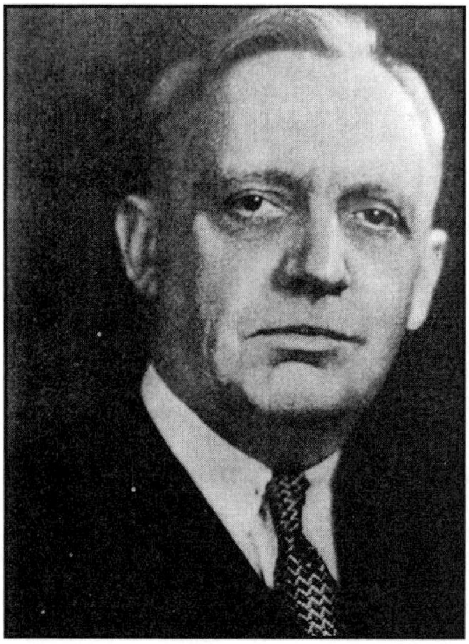

Dr. Ralph Carter
1884 - 1942
Photo courtesy of
Wisconsin State Medical Journal
October 1935 Volume 34

The 1934 meeting of the Wisconsin State Medical Society was held in Green Bay. Dr. E. G. Nadeau was general chairman of the meeting. The scientific and the House of Delegates meetings were held at the Northland Hotel and the annual golf outing at the Oneida Golf Club. Dr. R. M. Carter was Speaker of the House of Delegates. Clinical case presentations were given for the attendees by several Green Bay physicians. Fifty-three physicians from Green Bay, and a total of sixty-four physicians in Brown County were listed as members of the State Medical Society in 1934.

Dr. Ralph M. Carter was elected president of the State Medical Society in 1936. He eventually limited his practice to orthopedics (although he apparently never had formal orthopedic training), was a member of the American Academy of Orthopedic Surgeons and a

Fellow of the American College of Surgeons. In his presidential address to the State Medical Society he acknowledged the growing dissatisfaction with the delivery and quality of medical care to many in our country but was opposed to any governmental intervention. He agreed that there was a segment of the population that were lacking "in dental care, who have defective vision, who have infected tonsils, who need instruction on matters of hygiene; there are many children who need protection against small pox, diphtheria, and other conditions. But this is as much, if not more, an indictment against the people themselves than it is against the medical profession. Preventive medicine and public health measures are matters of education, and much ignorance, stupidity, and indifference has to be overcome. Can anyone who realizes the enormity of this problem believe that conditions will be any better under any system of state medicine?" Dr. Carter was a very strong believer that doctors should be the leaders in the delivery of medical care to the individual patient. He thought doctors should continue to treat patients regardless the prospect of receiving a fee. Dr. Carter noted "that we as physicians, are more interested in preserving and restoring health than we are in exploiting the people for our own advantage." A firm believer in the authority of the local medical society, one of his principles was "all health activities of the community are sanctioned and approved and under the direction of the county medical society, where they properly belong." [4]

One aspect of medical society control over the delivery of care was the fee schedule. The Brown- Kewaunee- Door County Medical Society published a minimum fee schedule for 1937. Office calls were fixed at $2; obstetrical deliveries, $25; appendectomy, $50; and tonsillectomy, $25. Physicians were expected to honor these minimum but could charge higher fees if they wished.

Despite the active role in Wisconsin and local medical issues by Brown County doctors, St. Mary's Hospital remained the only institution in Green Bay to have organized under the American College of Surgeons guidelines. The Bellin Hospital medical staff held meetings and discussed cases, but there was no systematic review of clinical practice. At a typical July, 1934 meeting preceding dinner, Dr. Walter Mueller presided. Dr. W. J. Decker reviewed a case of fever from a sinus abcess, Dr. W. Killins discussed a patient with heart block, and Dr. Hendrickson commented on a case of gall bladder infection. [5]

In October of 1936 the Bellin medical staff officially adopted the format suggested by the Manual of Hospital Standardization of the American College of Surgeons. Dr. Elverse Jordan, an internist from the Green Bay Clinic was the first president of the reorganized medical staff. The new standards mandated clinical record keeping including operative notes, pathological findings, and complications. Clinical conferences were to discuss complications, mortalities, and unusual cases. Other regulations concerned ethical behavior prohibiting fee splitting and the process of credentialling physicians for appointment to the staff. Appointment to the staff required membership in the State Medical Society. If approved by the medical staff, the appointment was then referred to the hospital board for final judgment. There was no credentialling of specific procedures or types of practice within the hospital. Physicians were free to do any procedure regardless of training. Accountability was provided by members of the staff in committee review of cases. [6]

The roster of the Bellin Hospital staff in 1937 included some new physicians. Dr.

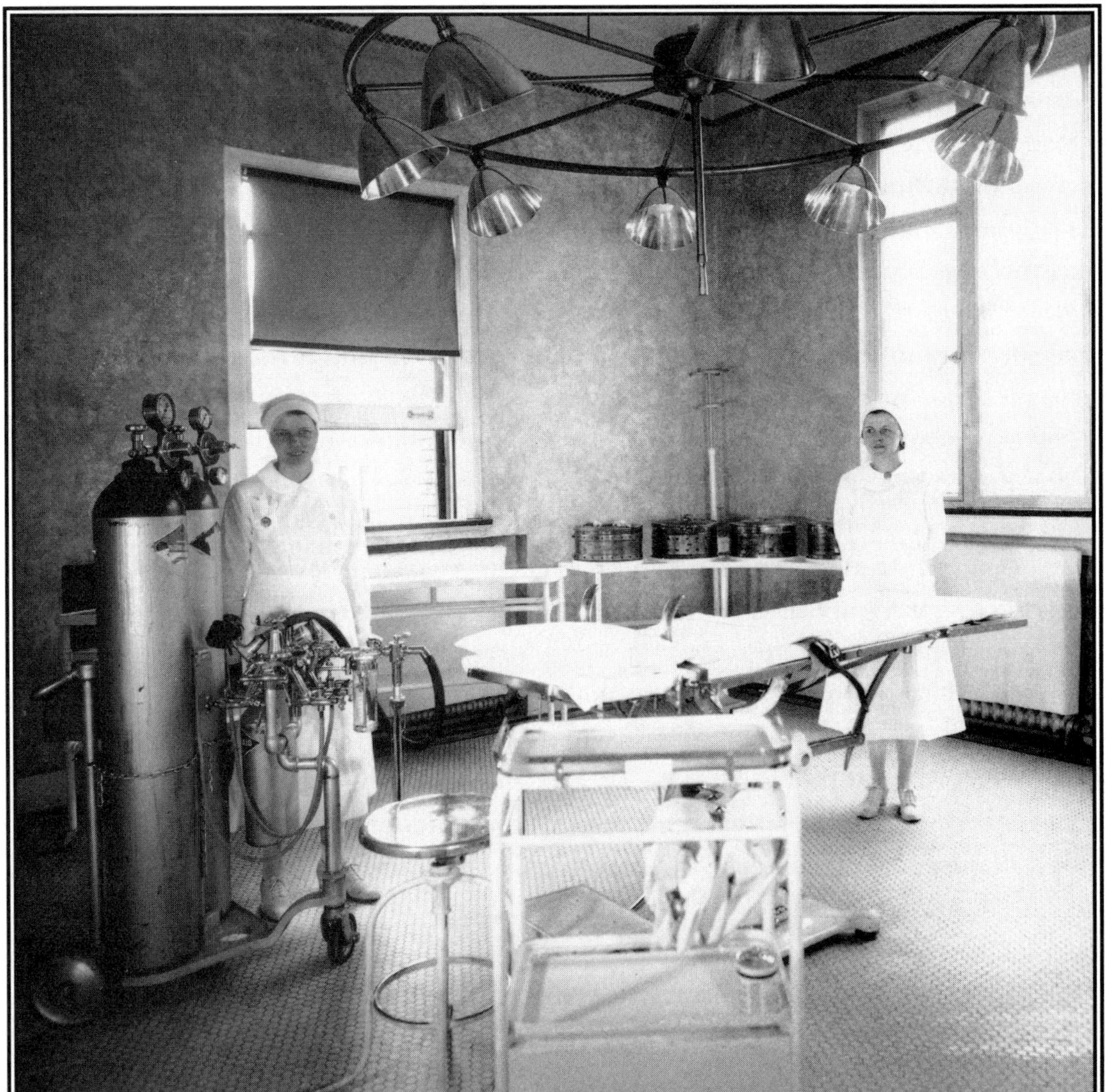

Photo courtesy of Bellin Health

C. S. Bolles, general medicine; G. M. Shewalter, radiologist; Dr. J. Vieux, general medicine; and W. L. Hardesty, pathologist. Dr. Bolles, whose practice concentrated on dermatology, was secretary of the staff. Dr. Vieux, a nephew of Dr. Bellin, practiced only a few years in Green Bay before moving West. Dr. Shewalter, a graduate of Indiana Medical School had been in practice in Kansas prior to arriving in Green Bay. He concentrated his practice in radiology and radiotherapy although he was not board trained or certified in either. His office was located outside of the hospital and he was not employed by Bellin Hospital. Dr. Hardesty did not remain at the hospital long and was soon replaced by Dr. Holly Heitzman.

At a January 1938 special meeting of the medical staff executive committees of both St. Mary's and Bellin Hospital, the status of X-ray and pathology services at the two hospitals was critically reviewed. Complaints of erroneous pathological reports, which were often late and inadequate were expressed. Physicians present at the meeting noted X-ray reports were made on inadequate films that should have been retaken and often two to three days elapsed before X-rays were even read.

A possible solution to the problem was suggested by Drs. Williamson and Troup. The physicians felt that the services available at St. Vincent Hospital were of better quality. They proposed sharing the pathologist and radiologist among the three Green Bay hospitals. [7] Apparently, despite the opposition of Dr. Minahan, St. Vincent Hospital had acquired the services of Dr. Jack Ford as pathologist and Dr. Steve Mokohrisky as radiologist in 1936-7. Sharing of physician services among the three hospitals would not occur. The arrival of Dr. Holly Heitzman, who had dual training as a pathologist and radiologist, resolved the concerns.

Dr. Holly Heitzman arrived in Green bay in 1938. He had completed a radiology residency in 1934 and his pathology training in 1937. Bellin and St. Mary's Hospitals shared his services as both radiologist and pathologist for many years. Before beginning practice he was an instructor at Tufts Medical School in Boston. Dr. Heitzman was a well read and enthusiastic scholarly individual who in 1957 introduced the Coulter Counter, an automated blood cell counter, to the area. Dr. Coulter, himself, visited Green Bay to introduce the advanced technology.

Dr. J. R. Minahan had achieved a very respected presence in the community due to his eminence as a surgeon and his many business connections. His legacy was greatly enhanced at a ceremony giving the deed to the Minahan Memorial Stadium to St. Norbert College's Right Rev. Abbot B. H. Pennings, O. Praem at a ceremony October 9, 1938. In the presentation, Dr. Minahan said, "I give you this deed to this land, and the building and improvements theron, free of all debt, that you may increase your college year after year, and send out hundreds of useful American Citizens." The gift was termed by Bishop Rhode "The brightest day on the athletic calendar of St. Norbert. The dream of many a year has become a reality. Many desires and hopes herein are fulfilled." Also present at the ceremony was Green Bay Packer Coach Curly Lambeau who praised the generosity of Dr. Minahan and heralded the event as contributing to the growth and success of St. Norbert College. [8]

The Sisters of the Third Order celebrated the first fifty years of St. Vincent Hospital with a Golden Jubilee dinner October 11, 1938. Speakers at the banquet lauded the Sisters for fifty years of service to the community. The perseverance and dedication of the early years were praised. Dr. J. R. Minahan stated that "St. Vincent Hospital is now as well equipped as any hospital in the United States." He noted the early days of the hospital and the ambition to make it a great institution and the fears of some that the new buildings and additions would never be erected. "And today I believe we need another addition. Green Bay has now been established for this whole territory as a medical center for this part of the country." [9]

Brown County Judge Carlton Merrill praised Dr. Minahan as the inspiration and force behind St. Vincent Hospital. "The result you now see before you was gained largely through his persistence and energy in those early days." Dr. A. J. McCarey, speaking for the Staff of St. Mary's Hospital, noted that physicians and administrators from all three hospitals were present at the celebration. His remarks would prove to be very prophetic. "All three hospitals here gathered around the banquet table is indicative of the new determination to work together in the common interest of the community. And, if that is done, our boast of having the best hospitals in this part of the country will come true." [10]

The Minahan influence over St. Vincent policy began to wane over the next few years. Dr. R.E. Minahan died April 27, 1935 and his brother, J. R. died January 22, 1941. The Minahan dominance of St. Vincent Hospital spanned four decades during which time the Sisters and the hospital prospered. Hospital capacity was 270 patients. Almost 8,000 patients were treated annually. Together, the Drs. Minahan and the Sisters of the Third Order of St. Francis had built the largest facility in Northeastern Wisconsin, equipped with state of the art laboratory and X-ray technology. Diagnostic testing included X-ray procedures, blood tests, bacteriology examination, allergy skin testing, electrocardiograms, tissue examination, and chemical testing of blood. The laboratory was staffed with registered technologists. A new physical therapy department was equipped with the latest in machines to delivery infra-red, ultraviolet, short wave, photo-therapy and indoctotherm therapy. [11]

The names of several new doctors appeared on the Bellin Medical staff in 1941-43. Dr. Fred Kuehl was the first allergy sub-specialist to begin practice in Green Bay. He was a graduate of University of Illinois College of Medicine in 1931 and continued his education completing an internal medicine program in 1934 and additional allergy post graduate work 1934-38. Dr. Kuehl was board certified by the American Association for Clinical Immunology and Allergy and a member of the American Academy of Allergists. Before coming back to his native Green Bay, he was the officer in charge of Allergy at Walter Reed Hospital in Washington D.C. [12] Drs. Ray Waldkirch, John Goelz, L. D. Quigley, Alvin Brusky, L. H. Sieb, Alvin Dupont, H. S. Atkinson, and Glen Denys, general physicians, entered practice in the area before 1945. Drs. W. J. Troup, C. S. Bolles, Carl Williamson, Fred Kuehl were called into military service after 1941. [13]

Hospital staff meetings and medical society meetings usually had educational case discussions as part of the continuing effort for physician education. What may have been the first more ambitious day-long program for area doctors was held May 23,1940 at Bellin Hospital. Films on brain operation, skin grafting, preparation of snake anti-venom, and the use of sodium pentothal for anesthesia were shown. A gall bladder symposium featuring medical and surgical diagnosis and management, abnormal anatomy, and a literature review of results of treatment was presented. Participants included Drs. Jordan, Williamson, W. Killins, V. J. Hittner, Ray Waldkrich and Louis Milson. Dr. Fred Kuehl gave a talk on the allergic state followed by allergic case reports by Dr. Bolles. [14] All presenters were local practitioners. Although this was publicized as an annual event, the war intervened. Thus another attempt to bring more formal continuing education to the area lost momentum.

In 1951, Dr. W. W. Kelly died. He was preceded by Dr. Fairfield's death in 1942. He was the last of the physician hospital founders to die. Dr. Kelly had many accomplishments including his guidance of St. Mary's. He was the Green Bay Packer physician for twenty-five years and a member of the Packer executive committee. In 1929 he was president of the organization. Dr. Kelly was president of the State Board of Health 1937-43 and was appointed a University of Wisconsin Regent 1938-40. [15]

Notes to Chapter 8

1. *Green Bay Press-Gazette*, St. Vincent Hospital Golden Jubilee Celebration, October 10, 1938.
2. Letter to Director St. John's Hospital Springfield, Ill., from Sister Superior St. Vincent's Hospital, Green Bay, WI., Archives Third Order of St. Francis, Springfield, Ill. 1933.
3. Stiennon, Oscar, MD, The Etiology of State Medicine, *Wisconsin State Medical Journal*, vol. 1934, pg. 710.
4. Carter, Dr. Ralph M., Address to the State Medical Society on September 19, 1935 in Milwaukee, Wisconsin, reprinted in the *Wisconsin State Medical Journal*, October, 1935 vol. 34, pg. 713-19.

5. Bellin Hospital Medical Staff Minutes, 1934-1936. Archives Bellin Hospital.
6. ibid.
7. ibid.
8. *Green Bay Press-Gazette*, October 10, 1938. Dr. J. R. Minahan presents deed for new athletic stadium to St. Norbert College.
9. See note 1.
10. ibid.
11. ibid.
12. Obituary Dr. Fred O. Kuehl, Green Bay, *Press-Gazette*, Feb. 20, 1974.
13. See note 4.
14. Program for 1940 Spring Clinic, May 23, 1940 presented by Bellin Medical Staff. The program did not include dinner which was seventy-five cents extra.
15. Obituary, Dr. W. W. Kelly, August 4, 1951, *Press-Gazette*.

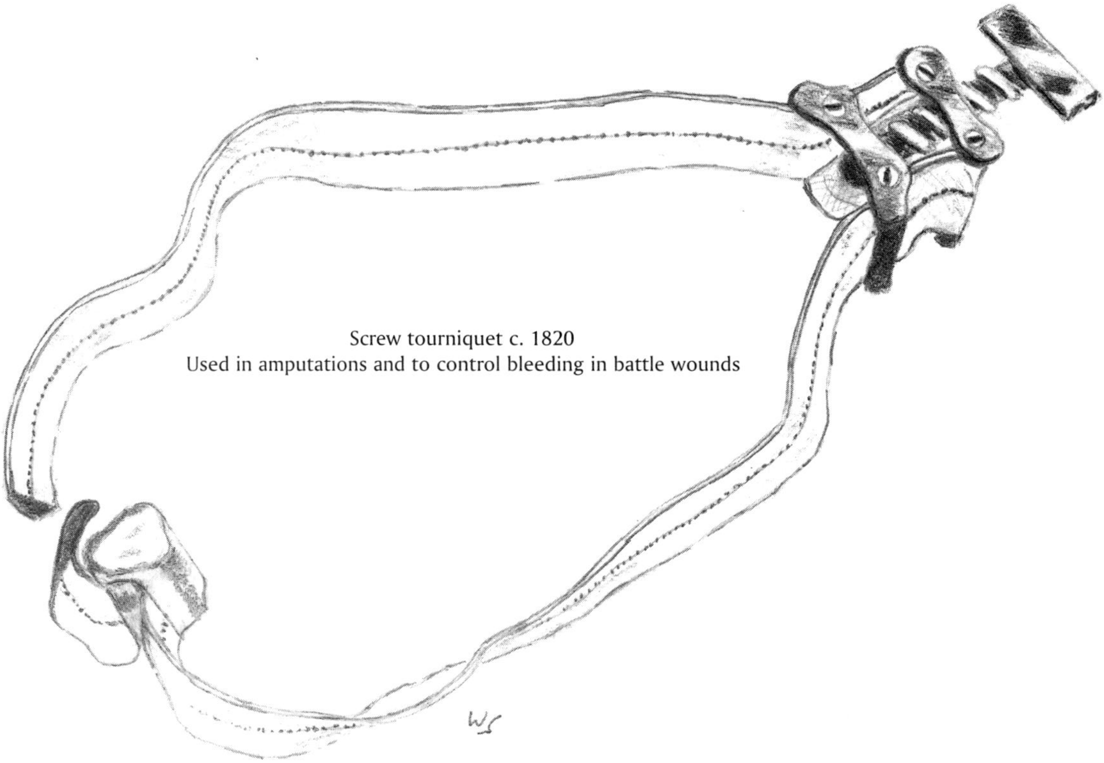

Screw tourniquet c. 1820
Used in amputations and to control bleeding in battle wounds

Chapter 9

Surgical Specialists

Drs. Glen Denys, Ken Denys, Eugene Brusky, Sam Brusky (Pulaski), Emmet Killeen, Ray Groendahl (Seymour), Ralph Lenz (De Pere), John Boersma, and G. M. Shinners, were listed on the Bellin Hospital courtesy staff in 1946. Active staff membership had been extended to Max Grossman, Al Freedman, L. D. Quigley, John Goelz (Brillion), and O. W. Saunders. Membership on the permanent staff was awarded after a year of courtesy staff appointment, supporting the hospital with patient admissions, and active participation in the medical staff committees. At the December 5, 1946 meeting of the medical staff, Dr. Ray Waldkirch, president, called the meeting to order. Twenty-four members of the staff were present. Dr. John Goelz was the secretary. The minutes of the meeting noted Dr. Milson read a letter from the National Research Council on the use of nitrogen mustard in cancer, Dr. Kaufman reported a case of probable osteomyelitis of the newborn, Dr. Grossman presented a case of ectopic kidney, and Dr. Jordan discussed a patient with a gall bladder problem. Four hospital deaths were also discussed. [1]

The Bellin Medical Staff reviewed the previous month's hospital mortalities at the

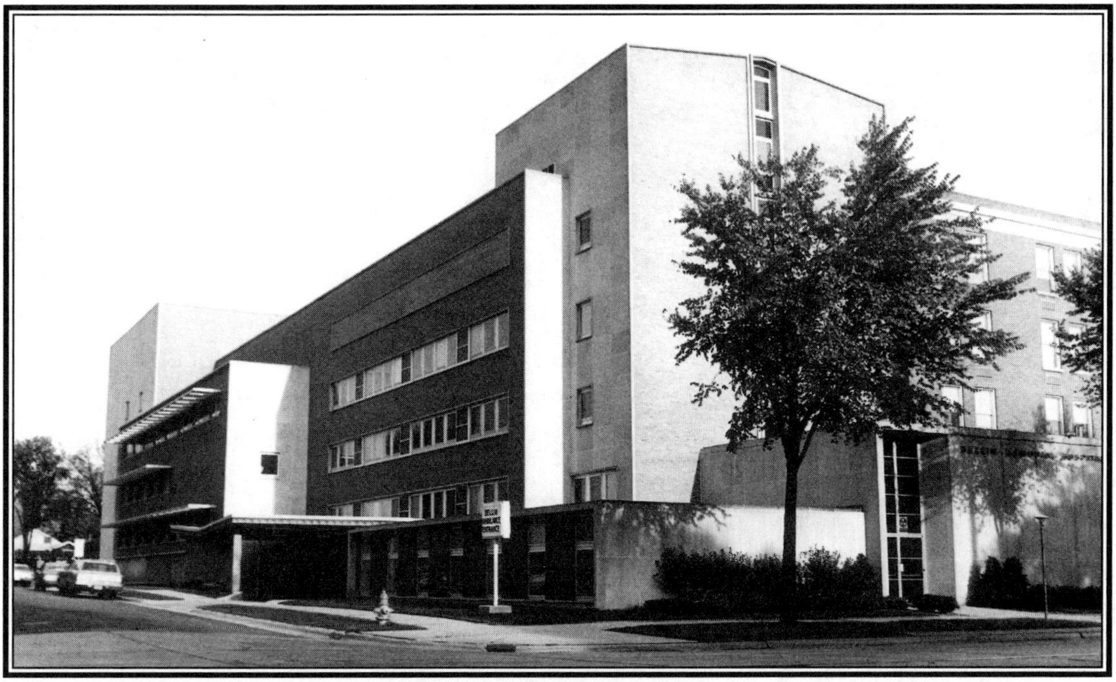

Photo courtesy of Bellin Health

December 1947 meeting. The causes of death mirrored the state of the art and advances which had taken place over the previous generation. Among the adult deaths recorded, only one was due to infection, four due to heart disease, two the result of cerebral vascular accidents, and two due to kidney disease culminating in uremia. One death was the result of an accident and the other from cancer of the kidney. [2] Antibiotics were dramatically reducing the mortality due to infection. Heart disease, kidney failure, and cancer were more frequent causes of demise in the hospital. The nature of the heart disease was just beginning to be better understood. Diagnoses such as myocardial degeneration and myocardosis were given to patients for lack of a more specific cause of death. Treatment of kidney failure by dialysis would not be available for another two decades.

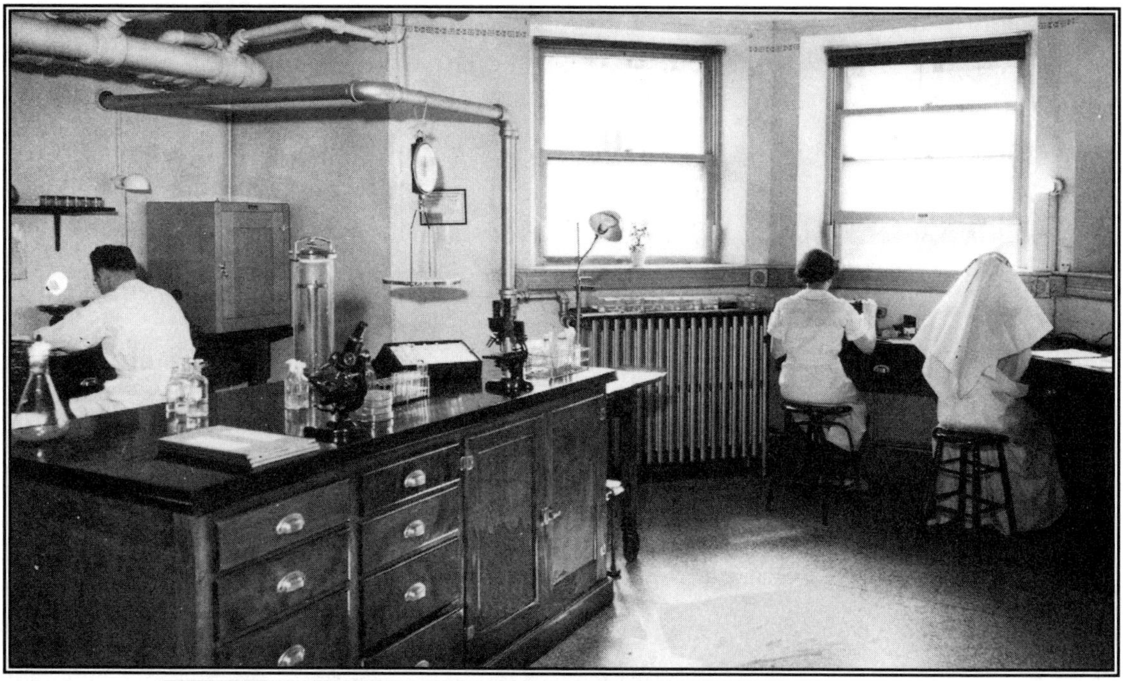

Photo courtesy of St. Vincent Hospital

The surgical committee of the Bellin Medical Staff in 1948 was concerned with the number of normal tissue specimens removed at the time of surgery. To reduce the number of normal appendices and gall bladders removed, a monthly survey of diagnosis was presented to the staff meeting. At the March 1948 meeting it was noted that twenty-eight appendices had been performed the previous month and eleven of these were normal or had no pathology. Of the eleven, five had been scheduled the day before surgery was done, thus calling into question the need for surgery. [3] The diagnosis of chronic appendicitis, at that time, was thought to be a cause of abdominal pain but inflammation of the appendix should have been present in the removed tissue. The more recently trained surgical specialists were attempting to change old practices and ensure that the accurate diagnosis of acute appendicitis eliminate unnecessary surgery.

Physicians trained in the specialties of medicine had arrived in Green Bay in the 1930's. The 1940 American Medical Association Directory listed Dr. Carl Williamson as the only board certified surgeon and Dr. Wendell Killins as the only certified internal medicine specialists. Dr. Ralph Troup and Dr. Steve Mokrohisky were board certified in radiology. Dr. John Ford had obtained board certification in pathology, Dr. Ralph Carter in orthopedics, and three men were listed as having board certification in ear, eye, nose and throat specialty. They were Drs. Emil Nadeau, William Comee, and Wilson Troup. [4] Dr. Albert Freedman and Dr. Jacob Kaufman followed Dr. Carter as doctors who had residency training and certification in orthopedics. Dr. Freedman received his MD from Emory University and his residency was served at University of Iowa. He came to Green Bay in 1944. Dr. Kaufman arrived one year later. Born in Poland, he immigrated to New York and graduated from Temple Medical School. After a twelve month rotating internship, a year of tuberculosis residency training, and several years of general practice in New York, he then completed an orthopedic residency program at the University of Iowa and entered practice in association with Dr. Freedman in 1945.

Dr. Max Grossman began the practice of urology about 1937 and was joined by Dr. Victor Neu in 1947. Dr. Grossman unfortunately became ill and had only a limited practice after 1950. Dr. Neu, Dr. Richard Troup, Dr. Ken Forbes, and Dr. Charles Smith, all residency trained, would eventually become partners in Urology Associates in 1959. They practiced in Brown County and held staff positions in surgery at the Iron Mountain Veterans Hospital and Dickinson Memorial Hospital in Michigan. Although prostate and kidney surgery was being done prior to the arrival of the urologists, better diagnostic studies and technical advances in operating procedures enhanced the treatment of genital urinary problems with the presence of the urological surgeons. Although competing for surgical cases, the urologists did not experience the difficulty in finding patients that the general surgeons had during this time. [5]

Physicians who had served in the military after internship, residency training, or who had been educated in the accelerated medical training programs began filtering back to civilian practice in 1945-6. Dr. Jack Killins, a Mayo Clinic trained surgeon joined the Green Bay Clinic replacing Dr. Carl Williamson who did not return to Green Bay after the War. Major Jack Killins had been assigned to the One Hundred Twenty-Seventh Evacuation Hospital at Dachau, Germany in May 1945. Medical observations of the German concentration camp inmates treated at the hospital were described by

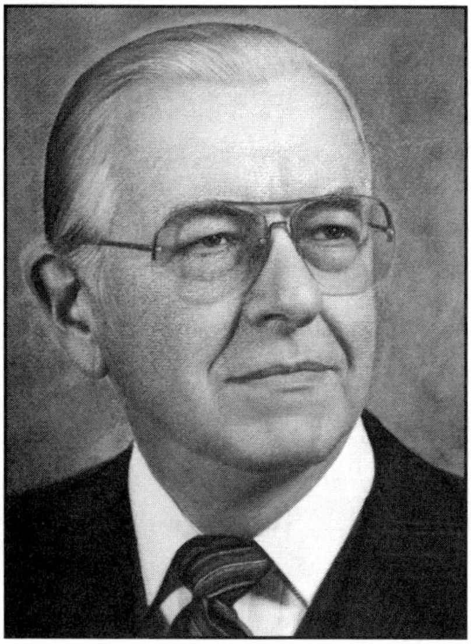

Dr. Jack Killins
1914 - 2001
Photo courtesy of
Wendy Killins

Dr. Killins in an article written for the Minnesota Medical Journal. Tuberculosis, skin infections, ulcerations, and general debilitation from lack of nutrition and inadequate sanitation were the most common problems. Tuberculosis was responsible for ten out of twenty-three deaths which occurred after admission to the hospital. Typhus was also prevalent, but suspected or proven typhus patients were all sent to a separate hospital. The experience would make a lasting impression upon the author as stated in the summary of the article. "The simple recording of these facts does not portray the sufferings of the patient's nor the unbelievable horrors of the camp. The human values are apparent, however, even in this factual report." [6]

A powerful new antibiotic, penicillin, was available to military doctors in limited quantities during the war. Penicillin was fast becoming the miracle drug for infections. The mortality rates of the United States military from pneumonia and meningitis was drastically reduced in WWII due to the introduction of penicillin. The exact indications, dosages, and routes of administration were still evolving during this time

Dr. Bernard Waldkirch was stationed in Japan after the War in the Pacific had ended. He was commander of a field hospital that had a low census at the time. There apparently was time to interact with the population. A fellow army doctor had become friendly with a local Japanese physician whose daughter had taken critically ill with erysipelas. Dr. Waldkirch had penicillin available but was under orders not to use any for the civilian population because of limited supply. After examining the severely ill girl and realizing how critical the situation, Dr. Waldkirch obtained the indicated penicillin for the desperate Japanese family. Administering a dose of 10,000 units of penicillin every four hours which today would be considered a low dose, the Japanese girl made a spectacular recovery within twenty-four hours. The grateful father gave Dr. Waldkirch several pearls as a gift of thanks for saving the young girl's life. After discharge from the army, Dr. Bernard Waldkirch joined his brother Ray in general practice in De Pere. [7]

Several doctors who eventually came to Brown County were involved in the military program to increase the supply of physicians available for the war. The Navy had the V 12 program and the Army the ASTP (Army Specialized Training Program). These were accelerated programs of learning partially paid for by the service and requiring payback years in the military. Among those who finished medical school under military obligation were Drs. George Hering, Ken Mickle, and George Crikelair.

Dr. George V. (Vosburgh) Hering settled in Denmark in 1946 to take over the established practice of his uncle, Dr. W. H. Vosburgh. Although Dr. Vosburgh had originally began practice in Cooperstown in 1896, he was recognized as Denmark's doctor. Dr. Vosburgh had practiced in the Denmark area for fifty years. Not trained in major surgery, he would often have to transport his seriously ill or injured patients to Green Bay for surgery. In the early years this was by horse and buggy and later by automobile. Upon his Uncle's retirement, Dr. George Hering assumed his practice. Dr. Hering maintained an office in Green Bay and Denmark for many years. Dr. Hering and Dr. Bernard Kulkoski had a busy Green Bay general practice. The Denmark practice produced some tense moments for the young Dr. Hering. Driving to Green Bay with an ill patient even during the late 1940's was a test of fortitude for patient and doctor alike. As a diversion, Dr. Hering's love of horses which he claims from his mother led him into raising and racing trotters.

Dr. Patrick R. Minahan served as president of the State Medical Society in 1946. At the annual meeting in October, Dr. Minahan referred to the escalating cost of medical care and the need for insurance to distribute the cost of catastrophic illness among many, especially the low income group. "Medicine contends that insurance should be voluntary as to the individual in keeping with dignity as a citizen." [8] He was emphasizing the Society policy of opposition to compulsory insurance by government.

One of the significant projections of the Society under Dr. Minahan's leadership was "to extend the scope of humanitarian legislation by appealing to legislative bodies to improve present hospitals and facilities for the care of the helpless and unfortunate. In conjunction with the county judges of the state, it is urging that all physically and mentally helpless be covered by appropriate legislation, leaving none, senile, paralytic, or cancerous, out of the program for efficient care." [9] Dr. Minahan's expression of self found in *Poems from the Annuals of Esmond* is consistent with his political endeavors. His poem "The Last Call" reflects the empathy felt by the physician called to the death bed of the poor.

A strong interest in local history led to Dr. Patrick Minahan's involvement and eventual presidency of the Brown County Historical Society. He died in 1953. [10] In a eulogy given to the local historical society, Dr. Oscar Stiennon eloquently praised the physician who had such a tragic beginning to his medical career. "Were we to write his epitaph it would be a simple one. His life is a shining example of gentle devotion to the cause of the sick. He sought not riches, not power, not glory but ever loyal to the ideals of his chosen profession, he walked humbly through his life doing good unto others, and died loved, honored and regretted by all who knew him." [11]

Just as Dr. J. R. Minahan and Dr. Julius Bellin dominated surgical practice in Brown County during the period 1900-1940, a small group of family doctors were able to do a large volume of surgical procedures during the next two decades. Drs. I.E. Levitas, Vernon Hittner, and Alvin Brusky were largely responsible for the continued growth of surgery in the area. Dr. Hittner did most of his work at Bellin Hospital and Dr. Brusky at St. Vincent Hospital. The surgical schedule at St. Vincent had a seven a.m. slot reserved for Dr. Alvin Brusky. Basically, all the general physicians were doing minor and in some cases major surgical procedures.

Dr. Alvin Brusky, a Marquette Medical School graduate, was the first of three brothers to finish medical school and begin practice in Green Bay and Seymour. Dr. Alvin Brusky supported himself during undergraduate school and medical school by his abilities as a barber. During vacations and weekends he practiced the trade, receiving twenty-five cents per haircut. One Saturday he claimed the Milwaukee record of eighty-five haircuts. He was able to pay for his tuition, books, room and board with the money earned as a barber. Dr. Alvin Brusky had an internship and a year of surgical residency at Milwaukee County Hospital before returning to Seymour and Green Bay. He soon established a busy practice, with daily evening office hours including Saturdays. Through his efforts, both younger brothers, Sam and Eugene were able to attend medical school. In addition, he helped support Dr. Robert Brusky, a nephew, and Dr. Dave Donarski, psychiatrist. Dr. James Feuring, an outstanding student at Seymour High School was also given assistance toward his medical degree. Sons John Brusky and James Brusky completed medical school and dental school, respectively, at Marquette. John completed an internal medicine residency before joining his father in practice in 1969. [12]

Dr. Leonard Miller opened an office in Green Bay in 1948. A graduate of Indiana School of Medicine and the Indiana University surgical training program, he found it difficult to find patients during his first year or two. In later years, when his practice was very busy, he would recall how slow business was in the beginning. There were so few patients initially, that he would leave the office by the back door and walk around to the front to see if there was a sign posted warning prospective patients to stay clear of the new doctor. A very respected surgeon and antique car collector, he and a twin brother were members of the Indiana state high school basketball championship team.

Dr. Harry Danaher finished his three year general surgical training at Milwaukee County Hospital after military service. His last year he was chief surgical resident. In 1952 he located in Green Bay. He would become the third board certified or qualified surgeon in town. Since most of the surgery was done by the generalists, establishing a practice was slow except for Dr. Jack Killins, who benefited from referrals through his association with the Green Bay Clinic.

The first general surgeon with thoracic training to arrive in Green Bay was Dr. Robert Wochos. His father and uncle had previously moved from Green Bay back to Kewaunee. Dr. Bob Wochos had spent two years in the military, passed his surgical boards, and practiced two years in California before returning to his native northeast Wisconsin. Dr. Wochos noted that the era of "personality based medicine was phased out" in the 1950's. [13] Green Bay had a reputation for "bad medicine" from the academic centers based upon alleged fee splitting, lax surgical standards and a poor academic environment.

Dr. Ken Zucker, nephew of Dr. Levitas, found it equally difficult to establish a surgical practice even though he had family in Green Bay and was board certified. Dr. Zucker graduated from Northwestern Medical School and received his surgical training at the Hines Veterans Hospital in Chicago. At first, he found himself doing general medicine and obstetrics to pay the bills. On one occasion he recalled being called to St. Mary's to deliver a mother whose baby was in fetal distress. The attending physician could not be located and the nurse called him in the emergency situation. Not infrequently, a patient would call on the surgeon to treat his respiratory infection and return to his family doctor to have his gall bladder removed. [14]

This was a time of transition for surgery. With the influx of well-trained general surgeons, the number of major procedures done by the family practice doctors was beginning to diminish. Many of the minor operations including hernias, appendectomy, tonsillectomy, and simple fracture repair were still done by the family doctors. Referral patterns remained the same as had been established during the Minahan-Bellin era. Patients from northeast Wisconsin and the Upper Peninsula traveled to Green Bay for surgery. There were not enough hospital beds and facilities to handle peak periods of use. In January 1948, the three Green Bay hospitals were full and patients were reportedly turned away. Contributing to the lack of available beds was the usual respiratory illness surge in the winter and more patients having insurance benefits. [15]

All three hospitals were making plans to improve and increase capacity by 1948. In June of that year, Bishop Stanislaus Bona of the Green Bay Catholic Diocese announced the first community fund drive for St. Vincent and St. Mary's hospitals. The goal was one million dollars. Additional funds to meet the expected total expenditure of three to four million dollars for the St. Vincent portion of the project was to come from the Sisters of St. Francis reserves and a bond issue. Bond indebtedness would also be assumed by the Sisters of Misericorde. Bishop Bona expressed regret that Bellin Hospital, which had already begun their own planning for a fund raising campaign, turned down an invitation to join all three hospital in a community wide effort. [16]

The Sisters of Misericorde, with community support, decided to move their Mothers' and Childrens' Home and Hospital to the West Side. They purchased property on Shawano Avenue in 1953. Reasons for abandoning the old St. Mary's for the new location were chiefly economic. The old facility needed extensive costly repair to compete with St. Vincent and Bellin Hospitals. Building an entirely new facility would enhance patient and doctor acceptance, and the West side of Green Bay was without a hospital and emergency room. A new hospital would offer conveniences for the growing towns served by Highways 41 and 29.

In 1954 Bellin Hospital opened a new five story wing bringing bed capacity to one hundred fifty. The new addition provided surgical suites, recovery room, diagnostic laboratory, and x-ray rooms. An emergency center was housed on the first floor facing Lawe Street. A x-ray therapy room was added in 1955. Bellin Hospital was the first of the three hospitals to complete a building program in the 1950's.

Polio was a dreaded disease in the 1950's. There was no treatment or cure. Physical therapy and rest with supportive care was all that was available to counteract the pain, weakness, and paralysis. Vaccination and prevention were just beginning to be accepted in 1955 when the height of the polio epidemic took place in Green Bay. Previous years no more than 32 cases of the paralytic viral disease were reported in the city. Before the end of 1955, 130 cases were recorded in Green Bay and 14 deaths were attributed to the disease. St. Vincent Hospital established a polio center to meet the high case load. Bulbar polio was not rare. At one point during the epidemic, ten iron lungs were in use simultaneously. School opening was postponed as a precaution until September 19, 1955. Fortunately, the number of cases rapidly declined by the end of the summer and the center closed November 7. [17]

Over the next five years, Green Bay would see further expansion of the medical facilities and a large number of new physicians entering practice. In many respects, a new era of medicine was about to take place. Larger and more complex hospital structure and function, a renewed interest in group practice, and more trained specialists would create a dynamic process that is continuing to change the delivery of medical care in Brown County and northeast Wisconsin.

Notes to Chapter 9

1. Bellin Hospital Medical Staff minutes, December 5, 1946, Bellin Hospital Archives, Green Bay, Wisconsin.
2. ibid, December 1947.
3. ibid, March 1948.
4. American Medical Association Directory 1940, section on Green Bay, Wisconsin Physicians.
5. Smith, Dr. Charles, personal communication.
6. Killins, Major Jack MC, Captain Joseph l. Posch, MC, Medical Experiences at Dachau, *Minnesota Medicine*, vol. 29, Jan. 1946, pg. 46-48.
7. Waldkirch, Dr. Bernard, personal communication.
8. Transactions 1946 Regular Sessions, House of Delegates, State Medical Society of Wisconsin, *Wisconsin Medical Journal*, vol. 45, 1946, pg. 1175-77.
9. ibid.
10. *Green Bay Press-Gazette*, Obituary Dr. Patrick Minahan, July 21, 1953. Dr. Minahan died unexpectedly of a heart attack at the Green Bay railroad station.
11. Stiennon, Dr. Oscar, letter dated October 17, 1953, to Wisconsin State Medical Society in reply to a request for an obituary honoring Dr. Patrick Minahan, former president of the Society. Excerpts of the letter later appeared in the *Wisconsin State Medical Journal*. State Medical Society Archives of Dr. Patrick Minahan.
12. Brusky, Dr. Alvin H., The Making of a Physician, Autobiographical sketch written by Dr. Brusky but not published. With permission.
13. Wochos, Dr. Robert, personal communication.
14. Zucker, Dr. Ken, personal communication.
15. *Green Bay Press-Gazette*, Jan. 8, 1948.
16. ibid, 6/2/48.
17. ibid, Dec 31,1955.

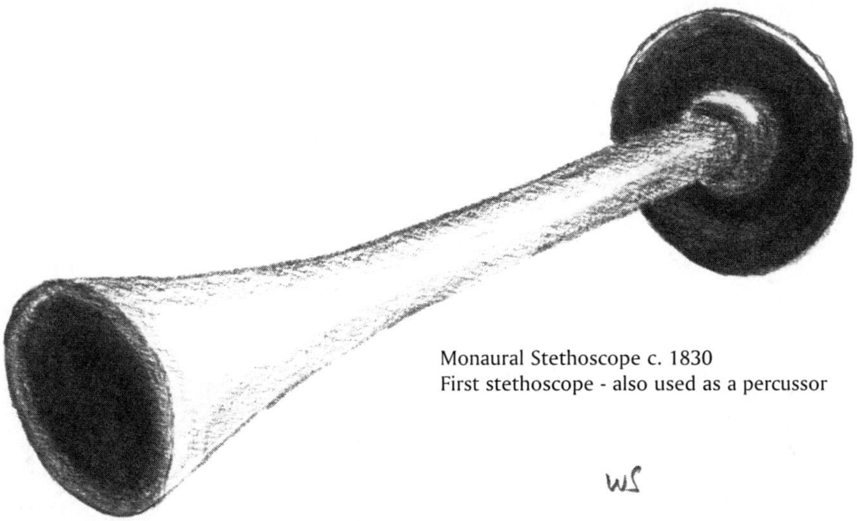

Monaural Stethoscope c. 1830
First stethoscope - also used as a percussor

WS

Chapter 10

Multispecialty Clinics

On December 12, 1957, the largest privately owned hospital in Wisconsin was dedicated in Green Bay. Bishop Stanislaus V. Bona of the Green Bay Diocese officiated at the opening ceremony of the new seven and one-half million dollar St. Vincent Hospital. The Sisters of the Third Order of St. Francis borrowed three million dollars to finance the project. The ten-story hospital became the tallest building in Green Bay. A five-story lab, x-ray, and physical therapy wing complemented the towering in-patient facility. Planning for the hospital had begun in 1939 but was interrupted by the war. A laundry and maintenance building to support the new hospital was completed in 1948. Construction on the main building had commenced in 1954. Three years later on December 12, the same day the first St. Vincent Hospital was dedicated sixty-nine years previous, Sister Canisia, provincial of the Sisters of the Third Order of St. Francis, expressed confidence the accomplishments of the past would continue. [1]

During the dedication program, Mayor Otto Rachals praised the work of the Sisters. "It is not easy to find words suitable to thank the Sisters for erecting such a beautiful building for the citizens of Green Bay. Dr. James Nellen, St. Vincent medical staff president, had kind words for the past and current superior-administrators. Sister Noel had carefully guided the building program to its completion before Sister Rose Marie assumed the administrator's position. Dr. Shinners, District Health Officer for the State Board of Health, noted the contributions of Dr. Jack Ford and the late Dr. Steve Mokrohisky in developing the "unexcelled pathological and radiological services of St. Vincent Hospital." [2]

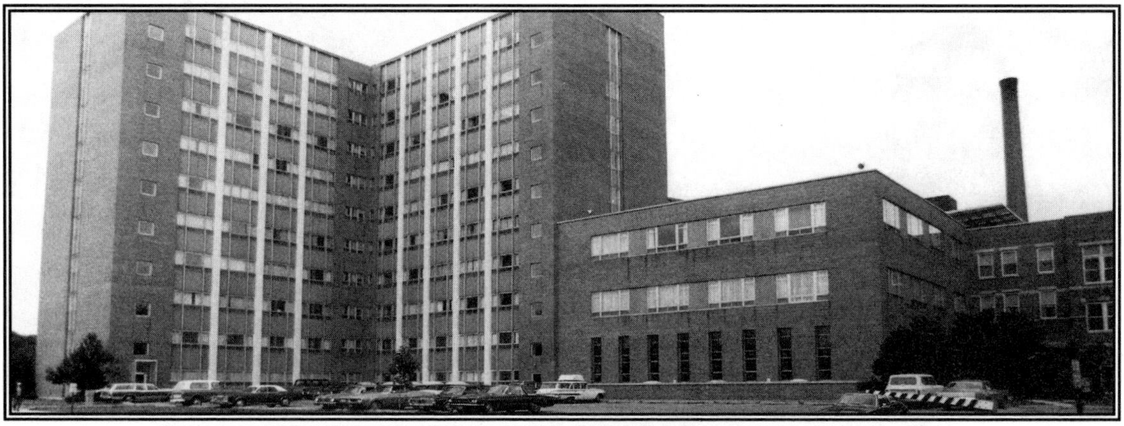

Photo courtesy of St. Vincent Hospital

The St. Vincent medical staff listed eighty-two active, seven associate, and eleven courtesy members. This included forty-three specialists and fifty-seven general physicians. General surgery, urology, orthopedics, EENT, internal medicine, obstetrics, psychiatry, and pediatrics were represented on the staff.

The opening of the new St. Vincent Hospital coincided in time with a change in the medical community. The family practice physician with one year of internship, and in some instances a few months of extra training in surgery, was still a majority of the doctors in the county. In the period following WW II most medical school clinical teachers were practicing physicians who had a dual role as clinical professor and private practitioner in one of the specialties of medicine. The effect of this was to enhance the role of the specialist and deemphazie that of the family practitioner in clinical medicine. The medical school professor often became the role model for the student. In addition, if the professor was doing research, he often encouraged his medical student or intern to follow in his path. Despite the growing number of specialists in the larger population areas of the state, Brown County was slow to attract internists, pediatricians and obstetricians.

The number of medical school graduates going into general practice was declining. The ratio of family practice to specialist doctor was rapidly diminishing in Brown county and Northeast Wisconsin. Many of the communities with smaller hospitals outside of Brown County were losing the family physician. According to the president of the American Academy of General Practice, the percentage of graduating physicians entering family practice dropped from seventy-five percent in 1931 to twenty-one percent in 1967. In his opinion the relative lack led to an increase in health care cost because fewer patients were treated outside the hospital. [3]

The gradual influx of trained specialists in surgery, obstetrics, internal medicine and pediatrics, beginning in the late 1950's would alter the delivery of health care in Brown County. The doctor that could do any procedure, treat any disease, or be the final answer to the patient's quest for health was being challenged by the specialist. Most doctors, recognizing the expertise of the specialist, were more than willing to accept the assistance of the specialist for unusual or difficult patients. A few doctors were reluctant to consult when faced with difficult problems beyond their capabilities. The more recently trained doctors often employed newer methods of diagnosis and treatment in conflict with older established medical practice. In retrospect, the older methods, and in some instances the new, were not always based on rigorous research. Because the established general physician had no restrictions on his privileges to practice, adopting the new procedures or treatment without adequate experience or training (in the judgment of the specialist) was a potential for poor results. This conflict between the old and new would be a source of continuing tension between specialists and the family physician for years and in a few instances ended in contentious meetings of the medical staff and administration of the hospital involved. The conflict would be settled only after extensive legal grievance proceedings proscribed by hospital staff by-laws.

Credentialing of new and present doctors to practice in the field of their training and experience began in each of the hospitals in the 1950's. Previously, a physician was admitted to the medical society and accepted to hospital staff membership. The medical staff by-laws of Bellin Hospital contained a provision that if a physician was not a member of the Brown-Door-Kewaunee Medical Society he could not be a member of the hospital staff. If he was rejected by the Society, he usually would not remain in the area. Rejection of membership in the society was a rare occurrence and was attributed, on at least one occasion, to the doctor's inflammatory remark that "only obstetricians should deliver babies."

The hospital administrator still had a significant role in who had special privileges as late as the 1940's. Dr. Alvin Brusky's growing surgical practice at St. Vincent was questioned by some of the older doctors but was sanctioned by Sister Rose Marie who informed the complainants "Gentlemen, I checked all the surgical records of all you doctors and I discovered that Dr. Brusky's surgery was better than half of you and just as good as the rest of you." Apparently the questions were answered. [4]

The medical society still had considerable influence on fees charged to patients. An active committee of the society met regularly with insurance companies to establish a "usual and customary fee" and at times resolve patient physician complaints related to presumed excess charges. The Brown-Door-Kewaunee County Medical Society published a minimum fee schedule in 1958. Although physicians did not have to adhere to the schedule, gross variances were noted by the vested parties. Compared to the previous 1937 published fee schedule, there were only small increases in non-surgical charges. A routine office call was only three dollars and a house call six dollars. Initial exam for a new patient was ten dollars. Surgical fees were higher. The fee for a routine delivery and care was $100. A surgeon could charge $135 for an appendectomy. [5]

Hospital Credentialing would eventually begin to erode the authority of the medical society in determining who would practice medicine in Brown County. Each hospital had, as part of its medical staff structure, a credentials committee which evaluated the training and experience of the incoming physician. Documentation of experience in various procedures, comments by his mentors, and passage of specialty board exams were all included in the evaluation. Obviously, a pediatrician would not be trained to do abdominal surgery. Board certified general surgeons had more training but less experience than the family practitioner who had done hundreds of gall bladder surgeries, but theoretically, the general surgeon was better equipped to handle the more difficult problems and the unusual. Internists would not be allowed to deliver babies or do surgery unless there were special circumstances such as assisting a surgeon. There was more concern with which specific procedures surgeons or obstetricians could perform. Not all training included every complicated procedure. This led to an occasional ongoing rivalry between specialists. More significantly, family practitioners that had been doing surgery for years wanted to continue doing the work that they had done successfully. In some instances, they were intent on doing new procedures or modifications of old procedures without the documentation of training or experience. Prior to creditentialing, a physician could attempt any new procedure that he felt within his capability, regardless of training. Although the specialists used credentialing as a means of protecting the patient, many established family practitioners, and in some cases incoming physicians, were angered by the perceived attempts to erode the physician's patient base and protect the practice of the specialist.

The first doctor in a new specialty always faced unique problems in trying to define his role in the medical community. Dr. Stewart Griggs was the first pediatrician to open a practice in Green Bay. A native of New York State, he graduated from the University of Buffalo Medical School and completed a pediatric residency at Milwaukee Children's Hospital before moving to Green Bay in 1949. Dr. Robert Cowles who had a very large obstetrical practice, encouraged Dr. Griggs to open a pediatric practice in the city. Dr. Ken Mickle joined Dr. Griggs after completing a residency at Milwaukee Children's Hospital and the required military service. Both pediatricians were board certified. Dr. Mickle recalled the first years were difficult because the children referred for care usually were very ill and often near death. Most of the patients they treated, however, were self-referred. At the time, St. Vincent had a pediatric ward in the old hospital which was run by the nuns. Often, orders from a few of the doctors had to be interpreted for specifics. This was especially true of parental fluids. The nun in charge would sometimes ask the pediatricians for their advice, or on occasion use her own judgment, on the volume and the time of parental fluid administration. [6] Training programs in pediatrics had equipped their residents with the knowledge and experience not readily available to the practicing family practice doctor. Drs. Griggs and Mickle were excellent physicians and soon gained the respect of the medical community and patients. Once pediatrics was introduced to the area, recruitment of additional pediatricians became easier.

Drs. Richard Myers and Dan Shea, Mayo Clinic residency graduates and board certified in pediatrics began practice in 1957-8. For unknown reasons they were not invited to join the Green Bay Clinic which had only Mayo trained doctors. Dr. Shea and Dr. Myers opened their practice in downtown Green Bay. Eventually Drs. Griggs, Mickle, Shea and Myers would be key participants in forming the Beaumont Clinic.

Coincidentally, Dr. Stephen Drake Austin, the first board certified obstetrician arrived in Green Bay. A native of Chicago, Dr. Austin graduated from Princeton University and received his MD from Harvard Medical School. He returned home for a residency in obstetrics and gynecology at Rush Presbyterian St. Lukes's Hospital. In 1953, he opened an office in the Bellin Building. [7] It would be six years before another obstetrician began practice in Green Bay. Dr. Herbert Sandmire who had his residency at University of Iowa joined Dr. Austin in 1959. The same year, Dr. George Theiler, a Milwaukee trained obstetrician, joined the Lynn Clinic, later to become the Webster Clinic.

Four more general surgeons would begin to compete for cases by the time the St. Vincent Hospital was ready to open the new surgical suites. Dr. Tom Lynn had finished a Mayo Clinic residency in surgery, Dr. Mason Letellier at Milwaukee Lutheran Hospital, Dr. Tom Beno at the Milwaukee Veterans Hospital and Dr. James Theisen completed his surgical residency at St. Lukes Hospital, Cleveland, Ohio.

Other specialties also saw new competition. Dr. Jim Nellen entered the practice of orthopedics in 1948. A graduate of the University of Wisconsin undergraduate school, medical school, and orthopedics program, he served in the Navy from 1942-1946 and was discharged with the rank of Lieutenant Commander. Dr. Nellen played football at University of Wisconsin and continued his interest in the game as Green Bay Packer team physician and member of the Packers Board of Directors. One of his many accomplishments outside the field of medicine was his appointment to the University of Wisconsin Board of Regents. In 1965, he was appointed by Governor Warren Knowles to a nine-year term serving as its president 1969-70. It was during his term of office as president of the St. Vincent medical staff that the new hospital was dedicated. He also served as president of the Wisconsin Orthopedic Society and Chairman of the State Medical Society's Committee on Handicapped Children. As president of the Brown County Medical Society, he proposed a third Wisconsin medical school be located in Green Bay. [8]

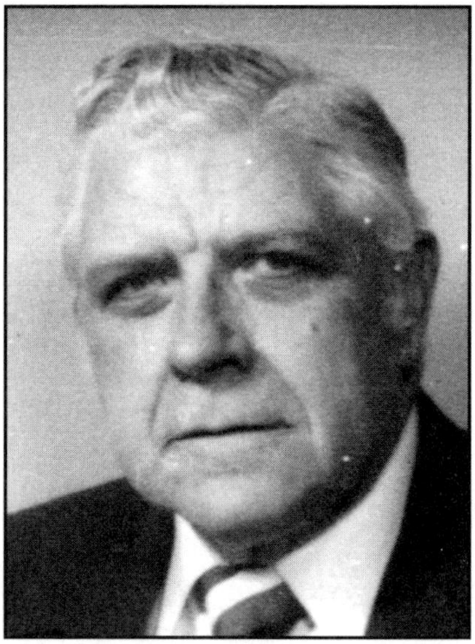

Dr. James Nellen
1913 - 1993
Photo courtesy of
St. Vincent Hospital

Dr. George McQuire moved his practice from Kansas to Green Bay in 1954. After completing Marquette Medical School, an orthopedic residency in Indianapolis, and two years in the army, Dr. McQuire practiced two years in Wichita, Kansas before associating with Dr. Nellen.

Dr. Eugene Clark, a graduate of St. Norbert College and University of Arkansas Medical School, started a practice in 1949 after a two-year residency in internal medicine at the Veterans Hospital in Cleveland, Ohio.

Dr. Joe Grace, a Mayo Clinic trained internal medicine specialist joined the Green Bay Clinic in 1956. He followed Dr. Wendell Killins and Elverse Jordan, both Green Bay Clinic members, as the third board certified internist in Brown County. The Clinic moved from their downtown location to Shawano and Military Avenue, citing the need for parking, more space and the growing West Side as reasons for relocating their office.

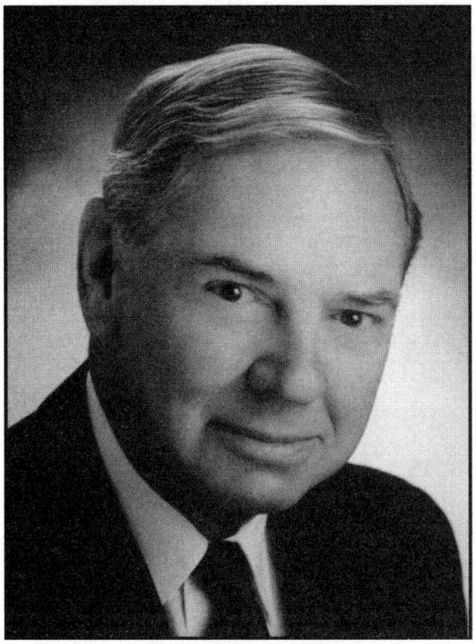

Dr. Joe Grace
1924 -
Photo courtesy of
Wendy Killins & Green Bay Clinic

Dr. Robert Johnston returned from three years military service as an infantry sergeant in Europe during WWII. After discharge, he entered Ohio State University, eventually graduating from the University Medical School. He completed a residency in internal medicine and hematology at Indiana University and the Lily Clinical Research Center. Dr. Johnston began practice in Green Bay in 1958. Initially, he was in solo practice but later associated with the West Side Clinic. Internal medicine at the time was represented by Drs. Wendell Killins who was nearing the end of his active practice years, Eugene Clark, Joe Grace, and the newest arrival, Dr. Johnston.

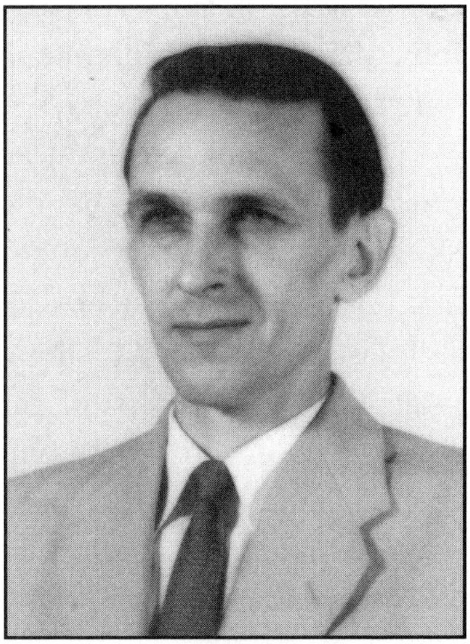

Dr. Robert Johnston
1923 -
Photo courtesy of
Robert Johnston, MD

The first hemodialysis for acute renal failure was done by Dr. Charles Smith and Drs. Joe Grace and Robert Johnston. The Service League had purchased a dialysis machine for the community. At the time, acute renal failure was treated by conservative measures and had a high mortality rate. The machine originally was rotated among the three hospitals but eventually was located permanently at St. Vincent. Richard Sandler, the first nephrologist came to Green Bay in 1974 from a renal fellowship at Barnes Hospital, St. Louis, Missouri. His stay was brief. Dr. Royce Lin, a native of Taiwan, was recruited to replace him in 1976. Dr. Lin received his nephrology training at George Washington University, Washington DC. Dr. Lin established the chronic dialysis service through St. Vincent Hospital and later what is now the Dr. Royce Lin Memorial Dialysis Center on Riverside Drive. The third nephrologist, Dr. John Lawton did not begin practice until 1985, before Dr. Lin's untimely death.

Dr. Marvin Blackburn assumed the pathology duties at Bellin Hospital in 1954 and one year later, Dr. Lyle Edelblute became the Bellin radiologist. Dr. Heitzman continued to do both specialties at St. Mary's Hospital. Drs. John Mokrohisky, Loren Thompson, radiologists and Dr. Ray McCormick, pathologist, located at St. Vincent Hospital in 1958-59.

Dr. (Sam) McCormick had been in the Army Air force in WWII. As navigator on a B 24 bomber, his plane was shot down over France in 1944. One of two survivors of the crash, he was imprisoned for ten months by the Germans. Returning to his native Wisconsin, he graduated from Marquette Medical School and completed a residency in pathology before settling in Green Bay. Dr. McCormick was chief of pathology for many years but was also well known for his editorials in the *Wisconsin Medical Journal*. [9]

Dermatology, as a specialty of medicine, was not represented until 1954. Dr. Philip Christensen came to Green Bay after Medical School, residency and a fellowship in Dermatology at University of Minnesota and the Minneapolis Veterans Hospital. Drs. John Marnocha and John Kenny, both of whom had their Dermatology training in Milwaukee would not arrive in Green Bay until 1966 and 1968, respectively.

Dr. Fred Cook was induced to become the first anesthesiologist in Brown County. Nurse anesthetists had been giving surgical anesthesia capably for years. New advances in drugs and the need for controlled oxygenation during pulmonary cases had led Dr. Robert Wochos to recruit Dr. Cook. In addition to his duties as an anesthesiologist, he was responsible for a new department of respiratory therapy at the hospital. Training for the staff and therapists was initiated by Dr. Cook and the internists. A certified Respiratory Therapist training program was established at St. Vincent under his direction. The role of the nurse anesthetist would gradually decrease but not be abandoned as many more anesthesiologists would arrive in Green Bay. Initially, the anesthesiologist worked with a particular surgeon wherever the case was scheduled, but as the economics of medicine evolved, the anesthesiologist was employed by a hospital and the surgeon assigned an anesthesiologist by rotation. The latter was a more efficient method but resulted in surgeons losing the prerogative of choosing their favorite anesthesiologist or anesthetist. Dr. Jim Mackey began the practice of anesthesia in Green Bay in 1961 and Dr. William Nicolaus in 1963. Initially, the anesthesiologists worked as a group in all three hospitals.

Dr. Richard Oudenhoven was the first trained neurosurgeon to enter practice in Green Bay. He opened an office in the Bellin building in 1958. Dr. Oudenhoven became proficient in a procedure known as articular rhizotomy. Dr. Robert Gruesen, who completed a neurosurgical residency at University of Wisconsin, followed in 1963 and Dr. Hiro Nishioka located in Green Bay in 1967. Dr. Nishioka was born in Canada and had his MD degree from the University of Manitoba and had a neurosurgical residency at Western Reserve University in Cleveland, Ohio. He was an Assistant Professor of Neurosurgery at University of Iowa before coming to Green Bay. Whereas his predecessors would eventually focus more on back and spine disease, Dr. Nishioka was the first to devote his practice to the broad field of neurosurgery, including surgery on brain tumors and aneurysms. Pneumoencehalograms and the radioisotope brain scan were the only localizing procedures in the early years of neurosurgery in Green Bay. When CAT scans and MRIs were introduced in the succeeding years both older procedures would be abandoned. Dr. Alan Wentworth, a Navy neurosurgeon with the rank of Commander had his residency at the University of Iowa when Dr. Nishioka was on the faculty. This association led to Dr. Wentworth joining his former mentor in practice in 1979. As was often the case, once the barrier for a specialty was bridged, the number of patients seemed to support additional doctors in that discipline.

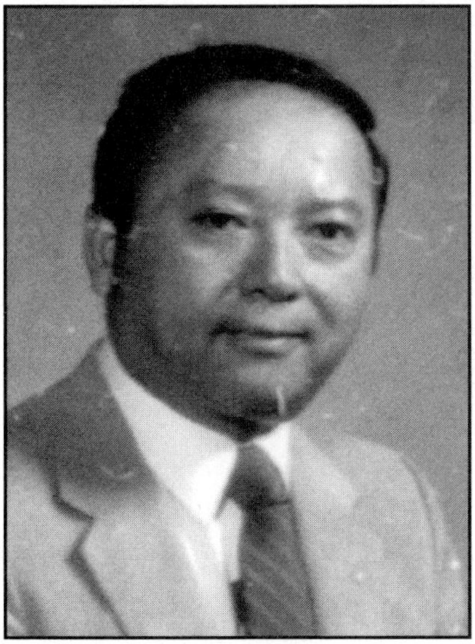

Dr. Hiro Nishioka
1930 -
Photo courtesy of
St. Vincent Hospital

Neurology was practiced by the neurosurgeons until Dr. Shamseddin Sarhaddi, a native of Iran came to Green Bay in 1973. He had completed a neurology residency at the Medical College of Wisconsin and was an Assistant Professor of Neurology for an additional two years at the Medical College of Virginia. Dr. Robert Schmidt, Jr. returned home to Green Bay in 1975 after a residency in neurology at Northwestern. One month later, Dr. Steven Somerville, also a Green Bay native, joined Dr. Schmidt. Dr. Somerville had his neurology residency at the University of California at San Diego. Within a short time a dispute arose between the neurologists over who was authorized to read electroencehalograms (EEGs) and electromyograms (EMGs). Dr. Sarhaddi, who was serving as medical director of the electroencepholgram department (EEG) at Bellin, was of the understanding that he should read all the exams done at both hospitals. Ted Jameson, administrator at St. Vincent was aware of the concerns doctors ordering the tests had about Dr. Sarhaddi's interpretations and asked Dr. Schmidt and Somerville to read the exams at St. Vincent. It was common practice for a new doctor with appropriate privileges to share in interpreting tests or procedures such as EKGs or pulmonary function tests. However, Dr. Sarhaddi refused a request to divide the reading of EEGs and EMGs (i.e. income) with Schmidt and Somerville. St. Vincent compromised by asking doctors who ordered the tests to choose who should read the neurologic tests. The result was not surprising. Most doctors supported the hometown men. Dr. Sarhaddi claimed the doctors and hospitals conspired to steal his patients and force him to leave town. Dr. Sarhaddi left Green Bay within two years but not before initiating a one million dollar law suit for damages against the other two neurologists and the hospitals. The suit was settled out of court for much less than the amount claimed. [10]

Although the number of family physicians entering practice was fewer, Brown County continued to attract newly trained general practitioners. Most did only minor surgery. They would do the more common procedures such as tonsillectomy, appendectomy and cholecystecomy. Drs. Chester Crawford, John Dettmann, Rod Erickson, Art Haines, Richard Jensen, William Schibly, and M. A. Warpinski were among those to begin family practice in the mid and late 1950's.

The Misericorde Sisters had participated in the community fund drive that helped fund the new St. Vincent hospital and a new St. Mary's. Their goal was to build a completely new hospital on the West side of Green Bay. Construction of the hospital was completed in 1960, and the old St. Mary's Hospital, a few blocks from Bellin and St. Vincent Hospitals, was closed and the property sold. The St. Mary's apartments now occupys the site. Patients and equipment were moved on October 10, 1960. Patients living on the West side of Green Bay who previously had to cross the Fox River for their medical care were now able to have their own medical facility, the first since Fort Howard Hospital. [11]

In addition to new facilities, new physicians and the influx of specialists, multispecialty groups began to form in Brown County. Aside from the Green Bay Clinic, most physicians were in two-or three-man associations or groups driven more by shared office space and sharing of personnel than by any medical practice innovations. The impetus for the clinics was very similar to the principles upon which the Green Bay Clinic was formed. Instead of going to several different offices for their medical care, the clinic could offer most services. Consultation and cross referral between doctors could potentially give the patient better care. Sharing of office space and employees was also a potential saving for practice overhead. Within the span of five years, five new multispecialty clinics were established. It had been thirty years since the Green Bay Clinic was formed and new clinics established.

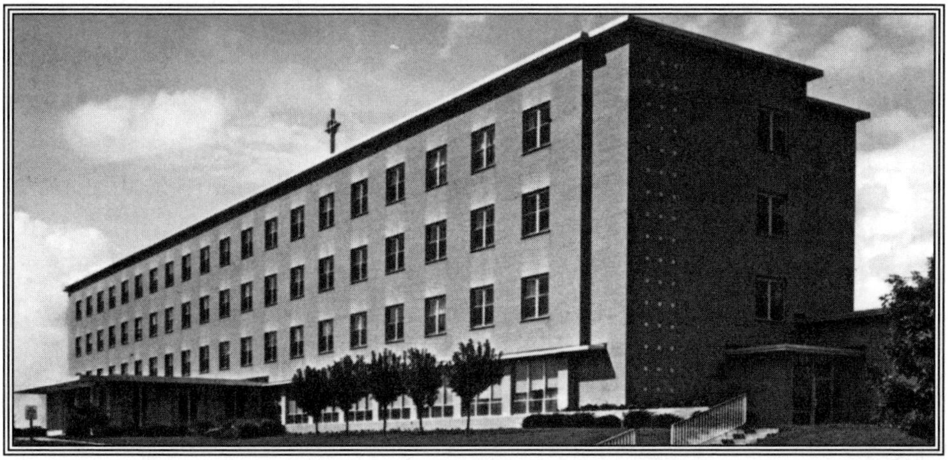

Photo courtesy of St. Mary's Hospital Medical Center

It is difficult to know the reasons why other multispecialty clinics did not start before 1960. The slow increase of specialists in the county, the recent success of large clinics in other areas of the state, and the trend toward physicians working together in the medical school and training hospitals may have accounted for the abrupt change toward group association.

Drs. John Goelz, John Dettmann, and Wallace Macmullen, family practitioners, were joined by Dr. Tom Beno, surgeon, to start the Goelz Clinic in 1958. Offices were located on Monroe Street just north of Mason Street. Later, this group without Dr. Goelz, would form the nucleus for the Deckner Clinic.

Drs. Eugene Brusky, Sam Brusky, Marion Warpinski, Jerry LeMieux, family practice; Harry Hoegemier, Robert Johnston, internists; and Mason Letellier, Bill Stoll, general surgeons; formed the West Side Clinic in 1960. The clinic originated at the corner of Gray and Mather Streets and moved to a new clinic building on Military and Dousman in 1961. The West Side Clinic would develop close ties to St. Mary's Hospital and eventually have physicians offices in the former nuns' quarters. The Green Bay Clinic, despite the proximity to St. Mary's Hospital, continued to admit patients exclusively to the East Side Hospitals.

Dr. Tom Lynn had become associated with Fabian Gosin in 1962. In a little over two years, Dr. Toby Theiler, obstetrician; Drs. Jerry Bramschreiber and Jeremy Green, internists; Dr. Roger VON Heimburg, surgeon; and Dr. Robert Kaftan, pediatrician, formed the basis of the Webster Clinic. In 1967 the facility was opened at the corner of Webster Avenue and Porlier Street.

The Beaumont Clinic was begun in 1962 with two pediatricians, Griggs and Mickle; surgeons, Wochos and Zucker; internists, Tom Leicht and John Randle; obstetricians, Austin and Sandmire. Within a short time the clinic added two more pediatricians, Drs. Shea and Myers.

Dr. Louis Milson, who was associated with Dr. Donel Sullivan, added Bert Milson, a general surgeon in 1961 and another son Stuart Milson, an internist in 1964, both trained in the Milwaukee County-VA system, to form the Beacon Medical Center. Dr. Don Gallagher, obstetrician, joined the clinic in 1966. The Clinic was originally located on Military Avenue and West Mason street and in 1970 moved to a site directly north of St. Mary's Hospital. It was renamed the Dousman Clinic. Members of the six multi-specialty clinics in Green Bay would compete with the independent physicians over the next thirty years before major changes in the structure of practices would occur. Individual clinics would experience growth of numbers even though there was a significant turnover of physicians within each group.

Another trend in practice association was the formation of specialty groups. The urologists had already established a single specialty group. Drs. Emil and George Nadeau and Robert Schmidt formed Eye and Ear Associates. Drs. Oliver Hitch and John Ottum joined to become the core of an eye group known today as the Green Bay Eye Clinic. There were three orthopedic groups. Drs. Kaufman and Freedman were first, followed by Drs. Nellen and McGuire. Dr. William Schneider began practice in 1967 and was joined by Dr. Dave Jones in 1969 and a short time later, Dr. Tom Kempken. The latter group, based in the Medical Arts building, were the first in the area to do reconstructive hip, knee, and children's spine surgery.

Of the family practitioners that came to Brown County during the 1960's, most joined one of the multispecialty groups or associated with a solo practitioner. Drs. James Falk, Pierre Slightam, and Jay Tibbetts joined the West Side Clinic. Henry Rahr went to Luxemburg with Dr. Henry Majesty, and Dr. Don Sherwood associated with Dr. Art Haines on the west side of Green Bay. Dr. Wesley McNeil became a partner with Dr. Chester Crawford.

A notable exception to the trend to become associated with a group was Dr. Darrel Angus. Dr. Angus, born in Oconto Falls, Wisconsin in 1927, graduated from the University of Wisconsin Medical School in 1949 at age twenty-two. After an internship and two years in military service, he completed a four year surgery residency at Akron, Ohio and came to Green Bay in 1956. Dr. Angus opened an office at 1071 West Mason Avenue. Although trained as a general surgeon, he did not confine his practice to surgery. In addition to his medical practice, Dr. Angus became active in city politics and construction.

The most dramatic change in delivery of medical care in Brown County in the 1960's was the passage of President Lyndon Johnson's federal government sponsored medical insurance for the elderly. Medicare and Medicaid, long opposed by physicians, became a reality in 1965. The other federal program which would affect medical care in the area was the creation of State Health Planning Agencies. The full impact of these programs would take several years to effect the delivery of medical care to the Brown County area.

Notes to Chapter 10

1. Cooke, Sister Frances M. O.S.F. Ph.D, *His Love Heals, A History of the Sisters of the Third Order of St. Francis*, Springfield, Ill 1875-1975, Franciscan Herald Press Chicago, IL.
2. *Press-Gazette*, December 13, 1957.
3. *Press-Gazette*, July 8, 1970.
4. Brusky, Dr. Alvin, *The Making of a Physician*, autobiographical manuscript written in about 1995, unpublished.
5. Brown County Medical Society, Green Bay, Wisconsin. Minimum Fee Schedule (for Private Patients) Schedule of Allowances Effective March 1, 1958.
6. Mickle, Dr. Ken, personal communication.
7. *Press-Gazette*, November 25, 1956. Obituary, Dr. Stephen Drake Austin.
8. *Press-Gazette*, September 25, 1999, Obituary, Dr. Ray McCormick.
9. *Press-Gazette*, Feb. 1, 1965.
10. *Milwaukee Journal*, September 15, 1977.
11. St. Mary's Hospital Dedication Booklet, Sunday October 16, 1960, Opening Tuesday, October 18, 1960. Archives Sisters of Misericorde, Montreal, Canada.

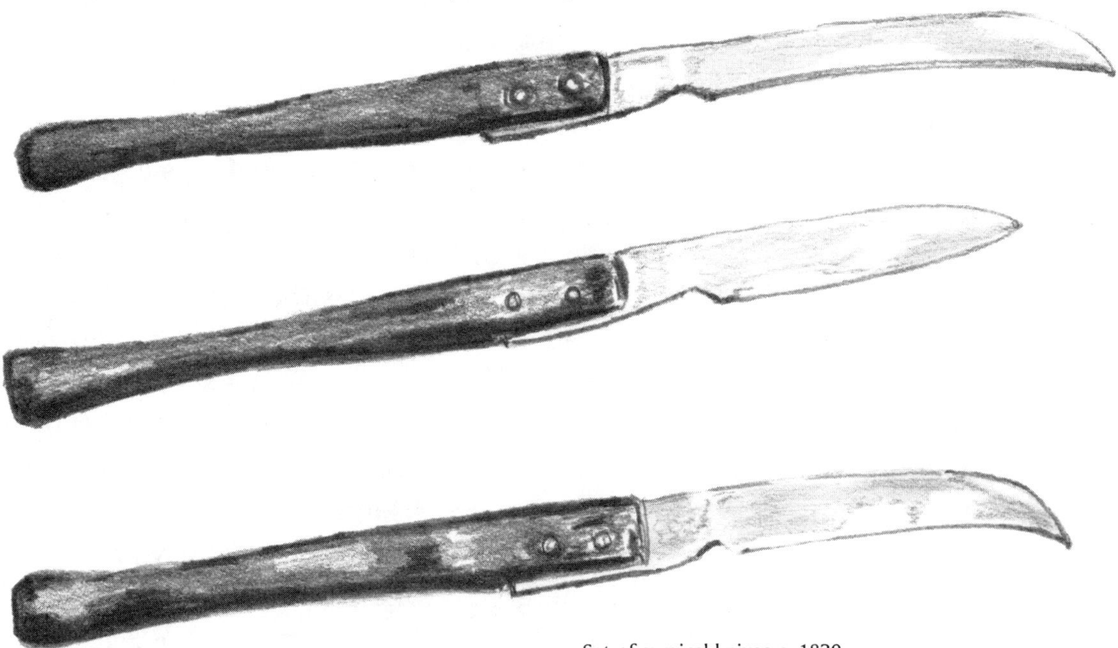

Set of surgical knives c. 1830

Chapter 11

The Cost of Improved Care

The 1970's were tumultuous years for physicians and health care in Brown County. The transfer of ownership of St. Mary's Hospital by the Misericorde Sisters, the escalating cost of medical care, attempts to curb costs by the State Health Planning Agency, a malpractice insurance crisis, and the beginning of managed care would be the seeds of a growing dominance of the hospital, the influence of third party payers on the patient-physician relationship, and destabilization of the independent physician and small group practice. In addition, the Supreme Court decision on a women's right to abortion and the new disciplines of open heart surgery and maternal -fetal medicine fueled the flames of controversy between physicians in Brown County.

The advent of heart beat monitoring devices (telemetry), new methods to aggressively treat rhythm disturbances, coronary artery catheterization, and open heart surgery led to the development of the cardiac intensive care unit within the hospital. The coronary care unit with its specially trained nursing staff had proven a major advance in reducing mortality from heart attack. The first coronary care unit in Brown County was established at Bellin Hospital in 1968. Drs. Joe Grace, Robert Johnston, and Jeremy Green, were instrumental in planning the four-bed unit. They trained the nurses to interpret cardiac arrhythmias and to respond to emergency situations. Only patients having chest pain or suspected of a coronary occlusion were admitted. Privileges to admit a patient to the coronary care unit were restricted to the internal medicine specialists and to any family practice physician who could pass a qualifying exam (given by the internists). Two family practitioners did qualify to admit their own patients. All other doctors who had patients with chest pain had to consult an internist to have their patient admitted to the unit. This was the first instance in which internal medicine specialists asserted control through hospital staff rules over the hospitalized patient and was initially met with resistance by many of the family practitioners.

The expanding importance of internal medicine specialists further eroded the family practitioners role in total patient care. The general surgeon, obstetrician, and pediatrician had already partitioned fragments of patient care from the family practice doctor. The patient now was faced with another growing group of specialists and possible loss of a traditional family doctor. The internist, obstetrician, and pediatrician were becoming the "primary care" doctor and fewer doctors were choosing family practice as a career, which only added to the expanding role of the specialist. Only two family practitioners came to Green Bay between 1968 and 1978.

In the summer of 1970, Dan Smith, administrator of Bellin, and Sister Valeria, administrator at St. Vincent, petitioned the city for permission to build a tunnel under Lawe Street connecting the two hospitals. They also envisioned a joint facility between the hospitals occupying a vacated section of Lawe Street. The purpose of the project as stated in the petition would be to "economize the community health dollar and provide the excellent facilities necessary to provide a continued high quality level of care." The joint facility was projected to incorporate a coronary care unit, cardiac catheterization lab, emergency room, and nuclear medicine area. The combined patient care units would eliminate duplication of expensive technology and personnel. [1] The City gave permission to vacate the street between the hospitals and the tunnel was begun but the combined facility did not have the final approval of the board of the Sisters of the Third Order of St. Francis. Shortly after the tunnel was under construction a new administrator was appointed by the Board of the Sisters of the Third Order of St. Francis.

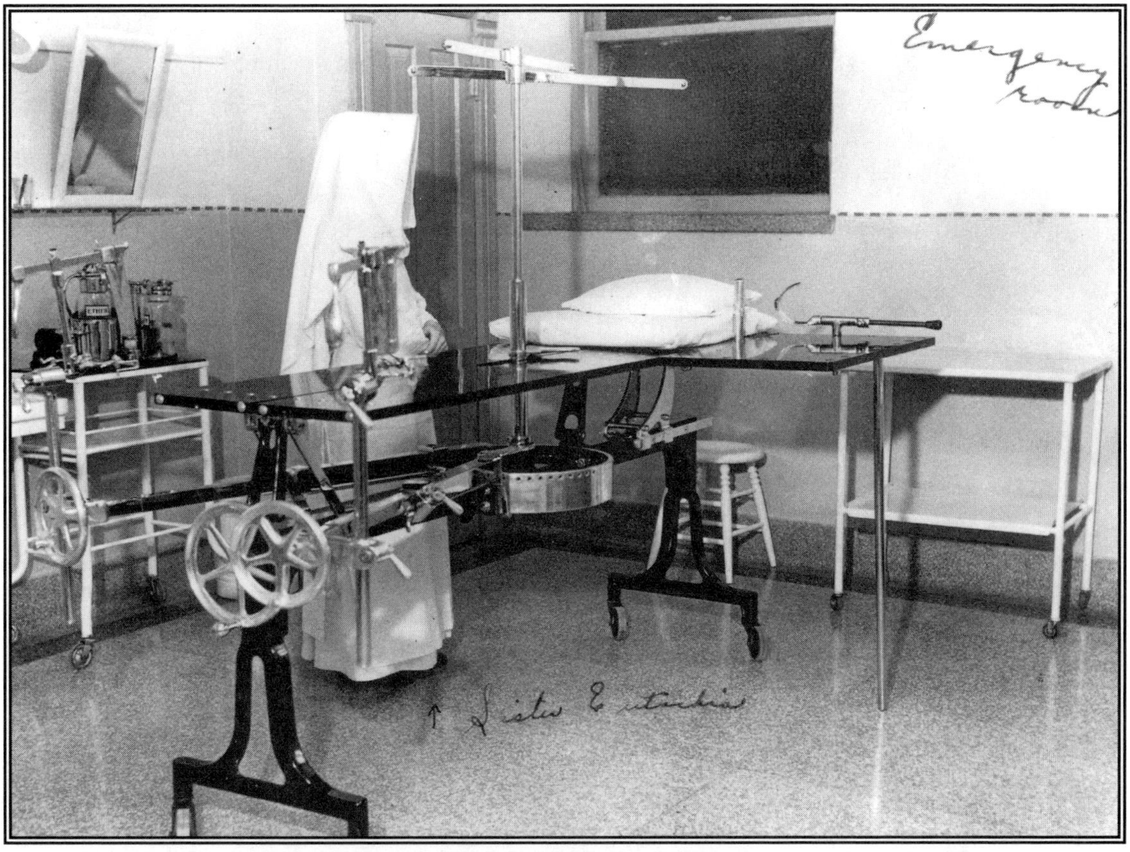

Photo courtesy of St. Vincent Hospital

At an August 1971 meeting, the Brown County Health Planning Council recommended that Bellin Hospital develop a heart catheterization laboratory and open heart surgery capabilities and that St. Vincent Hospital take over the responsibility for emergency room facilities. The intent of the recommendations was to prevent duplication of services and encourage cooperation between the hospitals according to Dr. Bruce Stoehr co-chairman of the committee. Sister Noel Bruseke, administrator of St. Vincent, registered the Order's objection to joint ownership and building a structure over Lawe Street but indicated the St. Vincent board would support the proposal of combined services if the need was established, the medical staff were in favor, financial backing was present, and all planning agencies approved. [2]

Within several months plans were approved by both hospital boards. Bellin launched a heart program to serve both hospitals and St. Vincent opened an emergency center for the hospital complex. Not only would there be cost savings in equipment, personnel, and facility but the need to have a minimum number of cardiac surgery cases to ensure quality was enhanced. St. Vincent built a new addition which included an emergency room facing Webster Avenue with lab, and x-ray facilities on the upper floors. Bellin remodeled the basement of the building on Lawe Street for a heart catheterizaton lab and used existing surgical suites for cardiac surgery.

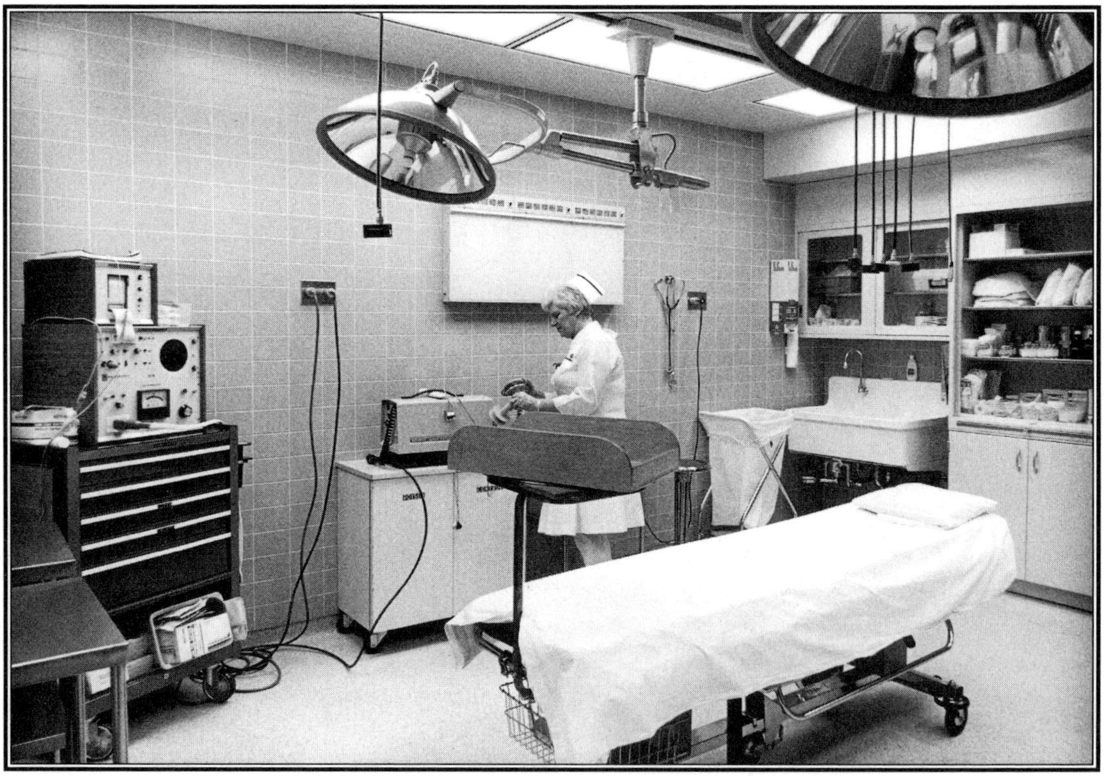

Photo courtesy of St. Vincent Hospital

The St. Vincent Emergency Center was staffed twenty- four hours a day for the first time by four family doctors who gave up their practices and devoted themselves to emergency room (ER) medicine. Prior to that time all doctors on the staff had to rotate through ER coverage. This obviously meant that expertise in treatment of emergencies varied greatly between physicians according to the specialty. Drs. Arthur Haines, Don Sherwood, Ray Groendale, and Francis Van de Loo formed the initial group which began working the emergency center in January 1970. "Our primary purpose will be to alleviate life threatening emergencies and to alleviate pain. We'll do immediate things, provide interim care until further care is decided," Dr. Haines stated. Noting the difficulties with the rotating system of emergency coverage he added, "The community is ready for this." [3] Most physicians welcomed full-time physicians in the ER as it meant fewer interruptions during the day and a reduction in trips to the hospital at night.

Dr. Howard Palay, a Milwaukee trained cardiologist was hired by Bellin Hospital in July 1972 as the first board certified cardiologist in Brown County. He was joined about a year later by Dr. Lewis Anthony who had his training at the University of Vermont. They were the first to do cardiac catheterization and coronary artery angiography in Brown County. Dr. Bill Stoll had done a few patent ductus operations and mammary artery implants without cardiac by-pass. Dr. Irwin Harris did the first open heart coronary by-pass graft in 1972. Dr. Harris was a graduate of the cardiovascular surgery program at University of Missouri and had been certified in both general surgery and cardiovascular surgery. Dr. Harris had been brought to Green Bay by Dr. Stoll in anticipation of building a cardiovascular surgical practice together. That association did not last long. Dr. Harris left Dr. Stoll's group and opened his own practice. In 1974 Dr. Robert (Jerry) Carlson was recruited by Bellin Hospital to provide an alternative to Dr. Harris. Dr. Carlson had his cardiovascular surgery training at the University of Minnesota and had been an Assistant Professor of Surgery at Cornell Medical Center before arriving in Green Bay. His publications totaled seventy-nine articles including many on myocardial revascularization. Amid controversy fueled by competing physicians and the hospital administration, Dr. Carlson moved to Neenah. Dr. John Soeter was invited to Green Bay. He received his cardiovascular surgical training at Vermont and joined Dr. Stoll's

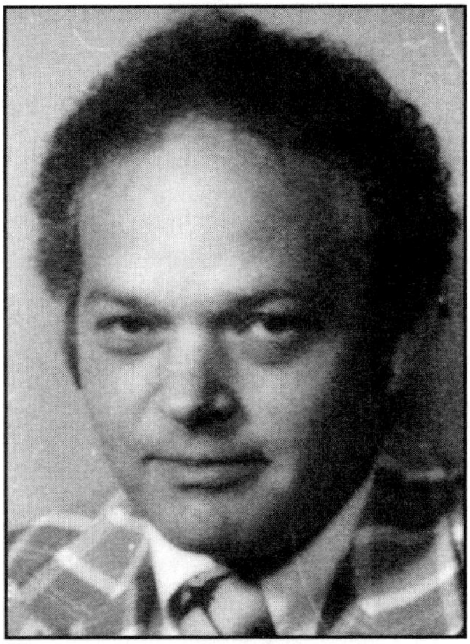

Dr. Howard Palay
1938 -
Photo courtesy of
St. Vincent Hospital

group in 1976. Three other cardiac surgeons practiced briefly in Green Bay during this period. For various reasons, they all established their surgical practice elsewhere.

In the first two years of existence the Bellin heart program recorded 664 heart catheterizations and 218 open heart operations. Four hundred eighty caths and 160 open heart surgeries were anticipated in 1975. The early success of the cardiac program was a reflection of the planning and the need for service in the area. Patients from all over the region were referred to the program. Much of the widespread knowledge of of the cardiac program at Bellin should be attributed to Don Gaetz.

Don Gaetz was hired by Dan Smith, Bellin Hospital administrator, in 1974. In four short years as director of media relations, he kept the Bellin heart program in the news with information which many doctors interpreted as blatant advertising. Despite the criticism of his aggressive approach, he remained energetic and no doubt was a factor in the success of the program. Fortunately, the cardiologists and cardiac surgeons defined success in healthier patients. In addition to his media blitz, Don Gaetz managed Bellin's fund campaign for the Van Buren addition to the hospital which housed the cardiac center; developed the multimedia Kresge Center; was the first director of the Bellin Foundation; and was the force behind creating Admiral Flatley Park in downtown Green Bay. Reflecting on criticism of his methods he said, "Bellin may have lost some patients and therefore revenue because some doctors may have used our public education program as a justification to direct patients elsewhere." His perspective on the business of running a hospital was expressed by "Bellin's three markets are patients, community, and physicians-in that order." [4] Physicians were reluctant to accept that order of importance.

Wisconsin began developing a state-wide Emergency Medical Service (EMS) in 1972-3. Each county and region had a committee of physicians, lay persons, and emergency personnel which organized a network of emergency facilities for the Northeast Wisconsin region and upgraded the transport of patients. Dr. Bruce Stoehr, a surgeon with the West Side Clinic was president of the Northeast Wisconsin Emergency Medical Services Council. Extensive planning went into facilitating transport of patients to the hospital with the best capabilities for emergency treatment of the patient. Dr. Howard Palay was instrumental in organizing and setting up the Emergency Medical Technician and paramedic training programs for the Green Bay fire department. The rescue squad would become an integral part of the medical scene. No longer would emergency patients be transported in hearse-like vehicles by marginally trained employees of local ambulance companies. The rescue squads were equipped with drugs and cardiopulmonary support technology and the personnel who could actually save lives in transport.

In a scene reminiscent of the old medical school amphitheater, the Green Bay rescue squad, accompanied by two technicians from Bellin Hospital, were called to the playing surface of Lambeau Field during the introductions of former Green Bay Packer players at a game in 1973. Eddie Glick, without warning, collapsed of an apparent heart attack and was lying on the turf in front of over fifty thousand football fans. Most were unaware of the drama taking place before them. The rescue personnel were called onto the field with their equipment (which included a defibrillator) and with the efficiency of well-trained medical technicians applied the electrodes to his chest. He was pulseless and not breathing. With one shock from the defibrillator, Mr. Glick was successfully resuscitated before the crowd could appreciate the dire circumstances. He was rushed to the hospital and lived for several years. Soon after this successful example of trained non-physician personnel on the rescue squads, training of paramedics and purchase of defibrillators for the fire department began.

The Wisconsin Department of Health and Social Services was interested in improving neonatal and infant mortality and in 1969 one of six regional neonatal centers was established at St. Vincent Hospital with pediatricians Griggs, Mickle, Shea, Myers, and Kaftan sharing the responsibility for a neonatal intensive care unit. Dr. Craig Anderson, who trained in pediatrics at Strong Memorial Hospital, Rochester, New York, came to the Beaumont Clinic in 1971. He would assume the title of director of the Neonatal Unit and with extra training became the first neonatologist based in Green Bay. Shortly afterward, planning for a perinatal center was begun.

The neonatal intensive care service helped reduce the neonate death rate from fourteen and nine tenths per one thousand live births to nine deaths per one thousand live births in the first two years in Northeastern Wisconsin. [5] This was achieved by the efforts of the neonatal intensive care unit but it was recognized that further improvement could be obtained by improving care of the mother who was at high risk of delivering a compromised infant. Even though Bellin Hospital had already developed a maternal high risk plan in 1974, Dr. Anderson applied for and received a State of Wisconsin grant to establish a regional perinatal center at St. Vincent Hospital. The perinatal center would include the neonatal intensive care unit and a maternal high risk unit. Dr. Fred Sehring was instrumental in planning the maternal high risk unit at St. Vincent. All obstetricians were eligible to work in the prenatal clinic and to have access to the nurses, dietitians, and a social worker to ultimately improve the mortality and morbidity statistics of infants of high risk pregnancies. Dr. Fred Sehring was appointed director of the maternal high risk unit and Dr. Dave Samuels headed the neonatal care unit. Dr. James Winston and Dr. Joe Brand soon joined Dr. Samuels as neonatologists. The St. Vincent Perinatal Unit served the Northeast Wisconsin District which roughly paralleled the referral area for the Green Bay Hospitals. Success of the Unit was largely due to the aggressive outreach educational programs, a well-conceived transport strategy which allowed for rapid transfer of patient to the unit, and very competent specialists.

The establishment of the Perinatal Unit at St. Vincent Hospital was significant for at least two reasons. First, the Northeast Wisconsin Health Systems Agency endorsed St. Vincent as the regional center and in effect declared the need for other centers unjustified. [6] Additionally, family practitioners, although encouraged to refer patients for consultation were not always involved in the final care or delivery of the high risk patient although in many cases the patient was returned to the primary doctor for delivery. This was yet another aspect of care lost to the specialist. Turning over a patient to the obstetrician because the patient had pre-eclampsia, diabetes or other high risk conditions improved high risk pregnancy outcomes but would further diminish the role of the family doctor in total patient care. Fewer family doctors already were doing obstetrics because of the high malpractice insurance for the specialty.

Almost all physicians consider malpractice insurance a necessity. In 1975 malpractice insurance rates were escalating and specialty physicians found themselves paying very high rates. Orthopedists, obstetricians, anesthesiologists, plastic surgeons, and neurosurgeons were charged up to sixty thousand dollars a year for malpractice insurance. The increase in number of malpractice suits and higher awards had reduced the insurance companies' reserves to unacceptable levels and the industry response was to dramatically increase premiums for the doctors. One group of Green Bay orthopedists indicated they might not see elective patients because their malpractice policy had not been renewed and they were unable to obtain a policy from other companies. In June 1975, Drs. William Schneider, Dave Jones, and Thomas Kempkin were notified that their "occurrence" policy would not be renewed by St. Paul Fire and Marine Insurance Company. St. Paul insured about 48,000 physicians in the United States and recorded a rise in claims from one in every twenty-three doctors in 1969 to one in ten in 1974. The average value of a claim doubled in the same time period. Predicted losses from claims in 1969 were $2,066,097. Actual losses were $13, 811,000. According to Clyde F. Schleuter, who was president of Wausau Insurance, the dramatic increase in losses paralleled their malpractice case experience with the Medical Society of New York. "The process has reached crisis proportions," he stated. [7]

The State Medical Society reacting to the concern of practicing physicians worked with the State Bar Association and legislature to solve the crisis. Physicians had threatened slow downs, early retirement, and simply quitting medicine because of the problem. A compromise bill to provide a state run medical malpractice insurance plan passed the legislature in 1975. The bill provided for basic insurance coverage of two hundred thousand for an incident and up to six hundred thousand dollars for a year's claims. A patient compensation fund for higher awards was also created. Both policies were based on "claims made." Claims made insurance meant that the insurer covered claims filed while the policy was in force. This was different from "occurrence coverage" that protected the doctor from malpractice claims alleged to have occurred while the policy was in effect, even if the claim was filed after the policy was discontinued. The claims made policy needed to be in effect even after the doctor retired and was to be paid by a lump sum referred to as a "tail" when the policy was discontinued. The lump sum due at retirement and the lack of restraint on pain and suffering awards were difficult for physicians to accept. The ultimate result of the legislation was to make coverage available to physicians for malpractice claims at an increase in premium to $80,000 per year for orthopedists, continue the dramatic surge in malpractice insurance premiums, promote an increase in the practice of defensive medicine, and increase the cost to the patient.

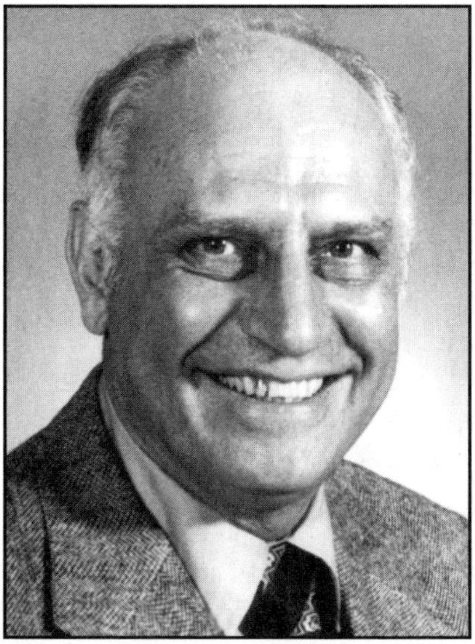

Dr. John Dettmann
1918 -
Photo courtesy of
Bellin Health

Dr. John Dettmann was president of the State Medical society at the time of the medical malpractice crisis. He had served as sixth district councilor for many years before being elected president of the society in 1974. His statement on the problems of health care delivery and financing was consistent with the feeling of most doctors. "Bureaucratic controls are not the answer, our experiences with government controls only confirm our earlier opinion that bureaucracy only exaggerates the costs and dilutes the services." [8] Dr. Dettmann also acknowledged the changes taking place in the practice of medicine.

"As we may recall with affection the valiant efforts of the old-time physician to cure illness and relieve suffering, we are inclined to forget how really inadequate his equipment and medicine were by today's standards. His skills, his concern, his willingness to give of himself were memorable, but too often inadequate to influence the course of illness.

The virtues of those physicians are still valid and useful today, but a great deal more is needed. The progress in science demands facilities and equipment and often a team approach to really serious illness. The changes in the character of practice are thus dictated more by progress in medicine than by a change in the character of physicians. Beneath the sophisticated exterior of today's practitioner is the less conspicuous but nevertheless still present sympathetic concern and dedicated physician who gives much of himself because he cares." [9]

The Federal government responded to the rising cost of medical care by instituting several programs which were designed to decrease the rate of increase in health costs and to improve quality of care at the same time. Medicare, which in itself, was a factor in increasing demand for medical services began to control cost by reducing physician payments and abandoning the usual and customary fees paid by the private indemnity insurance companies. A program to promote health planning for major facilities and technology was also an attempt to reduce expensive duplication and result in savings of the health dollar. Professional Standards Review Organization legislation was another law which was written to monitor individual practice pattern and reduce waste in Medicare and Medicaid insurance programs.

Wisconsin established Comprehensive Health Planning Councils which later were federally funded under Health Systems Agency guidelines. The purpose of the Agency was to control the rapidly rising cost of medical care in the state by eliminating the duplication of costly facilities and equipment. Each county had its own Planning Committee. Brown County was a member of the Northeast Wisconsin Health Systems Agency which was subject to the State Agency. This Agency would play a major role in the events of the 1970's.

The Green Bay Free Clinic was established in 1970 without initial support from the Medical Society. It was the only free medical clinic outside of Milwaukee in the state of Wisconsin. Several circumstances were unique to the time. The wide-spread use of street drugs, the anti-establishment culture of the Vietnam era, an increase in uninsured youth, and a relative high patient-physician ratio were factors in the development of the Free Clinic. The members of the Medical Society at first refused to believe that there was a population that did not have access through the system to health care but a survey of doctors' offices by Linda Pratsch of University of Wisconsin-Green Bay clearly showed that it was very difficult to see a physician if that caller was not an established patient of the doctor. Dr. Jeremy Green and Dr. Robert Johnston were early supporters of the Free Clinic and members of the Board of Directors. The community responded to the need for funds by providing a building and funds to operate. Robert Bush and John Brogan were key figures in a successful fund drive. Additional funding for the clinic was obtained by implementing the federal Women, Infant, Children (WIC) assistance program in Brown County which provided supplemental food for pregnant and nursing mothers and infants to age five who were found to have nutritional and financial risks. The Clinic also received federal funds from the EPSDT (Early and Periodic Screening and Diagnosis Treatment) program. The concept of the free clinic was to treat anyone who asked for care. Patients were triaged by a nurse and either treated by a physician who volunteered his services or referred to a list of physicians who would see the patient in his office for treatment. If the patient had insurance or substantial assets, a pro-rated fee was charged. The clinic became an institution in Green Bay and occupies its own building on Bodart Way at the time of this writing. The Clinic was run by an administrator and voluntary physicians. Laboratory exams were done without cost by the hospitals on a rotating basis. For over thirty years the Green Bay Free Clinic has helped meet the health care needs of a growing, diverse population which is without secure employment and insurance. [10]

The Brown County Medical Society was actively involved in attempting to control the changing environment of medical care and preserving the doctor-patient relationship and at the same time helping control cost. The Society investigated several prepaid insurance plans for Brown County, hoping to prevent insurance company owned and administered managed care plans from gaining a foothold in the area. The threat of an insurance company determining prepaid fees, developing closed panels of physicians, and controlling physicians' practices motivated the Society to act. The Green Bay Health Protection Plan was the final result. A cooperative venture with Wausau Insurance, physicians of Brown County, and the three Green Bay Hospitals was launched January 1973. The unique features of the plan were that any doctor could sign up, the doctors shared in the risk for patient services on a fee for service basis. If the patient fund was short, the physicians were charged and if there was an excess, the physicians profited. Similarly, if hospital expenses were less than the hospital fund pool, the surplus would go back to the physician, hospital, and consumer. In addition, physician review committees monitored physician fees and patient care. The patients were rewarded with better office and preventive care insurance benefits. In spite of the obvious benefits of the plan, there were many physicians opposed. Not all would sign on as participants. In fact, at the April 1973 meeting of the Medical Society, four months after the plan was in effect, a motion was passed to notify the media that the Brown County Medical Society was opposed to the Green Bay Health Protection Plan (Red Apple Plan). Despite the vote, the Plan went ahead and the majority of physicians in the Society were participants. Members appointed by the Brown County Medical Society served on the peer review committees. [11] The Red Apple Plan did bring a prepaid health plan to the area that initially was able to reduce the rapidly rising cost of health insurance. Eventually, however, higher cost and ever increasing control by the insurance company doomed the plan.

In January 1973, abortion became legal in the United States. The governing boards of St. Vincent's and St. Mary's Hospitals, both private hospitals, accepted the Catholic Hospital code and did not permit abortions in their hospitals. The Methodist affiliated Bellin Hospital Board and Medical Staff had adopted a policy of permitting an abortion only when the mother's health was in danger. The attending doctor also was required to obtain consultation with two physicians who were in agreement before the procedure could be performed. This policy was more restrictive than state law. [12]

Dr. Herbert Sandmire sued Bellin Hospital in United States District Court in April 1973 claiming his patient was denied her legal right to have a first trimester abortion at Bellin. Dr. Sandmire's attorney argued that since Bellin Hospital had received federal Hill Burton funds, it was a state hospital and could not refuse permission for a procedure legalized by the United States Supreme Court. [13] District Court Judge, Myron Gordon, agreed with Dr. Sandmire but Bellin Hospital appealed to the Circuit Court of Appeals and received a stay. On appeal, the case quickly went to the United States Supreme Court and in a seven to nothing opinion, the Supreme Court agreed with the Circuit Court and eventually Judge Gordon's initial ruling was overturned, reaffirming Bellin as a private institution and the hospital board's right to determine its own abortion policy. [14] This was an important decision because it gave the private hospital board added authority over physician-patient care and at the same time increased its responsibility for care of patients.

Dr. Sandmire, firmly believed he should be allowed to provide complete obstetrical care to his patients. Prevention of maternal morbidity from abortion procedures done by untrained practitioners was one of the major reasons for his support of the Supreme Court decision on a woman's right to have an abortion. At the same time, he was a proponent of the birth control pill and was active in establishing Planned Parenthood in Green Bay. Because of differences of opinion concerning the abortion issue and other financial aspects of practice, Dr. Sandmire and Austin left the Beaumont Clinic in August 1973, shortly after the refusal of Bellin to allow abortions in the hospital except under the strictest conditions.

Bellin Hospital initiated the building of a Doctors' office condominium just north of the hospital in response to a growing need for specialist offices located near the hospital. Drs. Sandmire and Austin purchased office space on the third floor. They were soon joined by Dr. Richard Bechtel, a graduate of Duke University Medical School and the Blodgett Memorial Hospital Obstetrical Residency program, Grand Rapids, Michigan.

Brown County was not immune to the rising cost of medical care at the time. One of the developing trends in the country was to reduce the cost of surgery by performing minor surgery in free-standing surgery centers. This could eliminate the need for expense related to many of the higher cost of care in a full service hospital requiring twenty-four-hour-a-day personnel. The Green Bay Surgery Center, the first out-patient surgery center not affiliated with a hospital, was opened in January 1978 by Drs. Sandmire, Austin, Bechtel, and Harold Hoops, plastic surgeon. It was located on the third floor of the Medical Arts Condominium. The benefits of the concept were immediately apparent. Procedures could be performed at a significant reduction in cost compared to identical procedures done in the hospital. Also the abortion policy was not subject to the hospital board. It was generally accepted that abortions were performed in the building leading to protest picketing and on one occasion a bomb threat to the Medical Arts building.

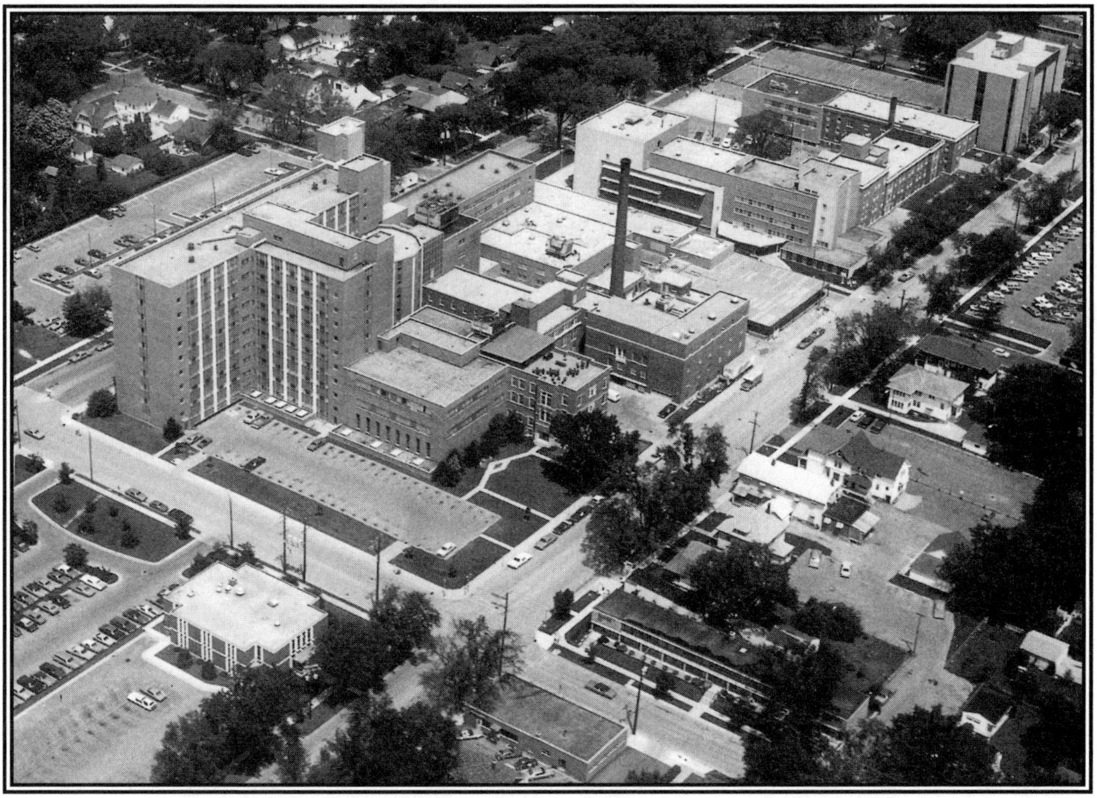

Photo courtesy of Bellin Health

Notable events were transpiring on the West side of Green Bay during this time. St. Mary's Hospital was for sale in 1973. The Sisters of Misericorde "lacked sufficient religious personnel who were committed to hospital service and running the hospital was not the main objective of the Order" according to Mother Superior Clemence Brabant. In addition, the Order wanted to relinquish its hospitals and pursue other objectives. [15]

Dan Smith, administrator of Bellin Hospital made an offer for the hospital which was very close to acceptance but at the last minute, Bishop Aloysis Wycislo of the Green Bay Diocese said that according to canon law the Misericorde Order must have Vatican approval to dispose of Catholic Church property. Acting as an intermediary for the sisters, the bishop had referred the request for sale of St. Mary's to Bellin directly to the Vatican. "Not even a bishop can do it without permission," noted Bishop Wycislo. [16]

Three months later, the Third Order of St. Francis Sisters agreed to operate the hospital. Bishop Wycislo was unsuccessful in finding an alternative buyer. The "sale" of St. Mary's did not come under health planning jurisdiction because the unusual transaction was finalized as a continuation of the St. Mary's Hospital Medical Center of Green Bay, Incorporated. "There is no sale. There is no transfer. There is no transfer of money. There is no donation of assets." stated Lloyd Planert attorney for the Sister of The Third Order. It was pointed out that St. Mary's would become one of twelve hospitals operated by the Third Order of St. Francis and be independent of St. Vincent. [17] On July 2, 1974 a new board of directors for St. Mary's was elected. The board was chaired by Sister Mariana Kosior of the Third Order and included four additional Sisters from the Order, Sister Rainville of the Misericorde Order, and two lay members from the community. [18] There would be no health planning review of the change in control of the hospital because legally there was no expenditure of funds over one hundred thousand dollars, the criteria requiring review established by state law.

The acquisition of St. Mary's Hospital by the Sisters of the Third Order of St. Francis would eventually dictate a course of continuing expansion of Bellin Hospital in the location directly adjacent to St. Vincent. St. Mary's would remain a smaller facility. Most referral patients were treated at the East side complex where the majority of specialists practiced. As the population of Brown County has grown and the St. Vincent Bellin medical complex has expanded, many in the medical community have speculated on the course of events if Bellin had purchased St. Mary's and Green Bay had East Side and West Side full service hospital centers.

It was not long before planning began on a entirely new St. Mary's Hospital. The original hospital was underfunded and architectural adjustments were made to meet budget. Room width had been reduced by one foot at the time of construction, the bed capacity was not considered optimum for cost effectiveness, and the foundation would not support additional floors according to architects Berners, Schober, and Kilp. The new facility was projected to cost twenty million dollars. This amount would be the largest sum to be used for hospital construction in the history of Brown County. Before it could be built, however, the proposal had to be approved by county, regional, and state Health Systems agencies. The Brown County Agency voted in favor of the project but the regional Health Systems Agency voted against the proposal by a close vote. The high cost and additional hospital beds planned were reasons given as objections. The State Division of Health and Social Services overturned the regional committee decision in March 1978 and approved construction of the new St. Mary's Hospital with a reduction in beds from 184 to 158, and one less floor. [19] A need for more beds at St. Mary's, inadequate square footage for the projected utilization, inability to meet standards and current codes for hospitals, high cost of remodeling the existing structure, and the need for a hospital to serve the Western area of the county were reasons given for the State Division of Health and Social Services reversal of the regional planning committee decision. [20] The new structure was completed in November 16, 1981. The old hospital was converted to doctors offices and administrative offices.

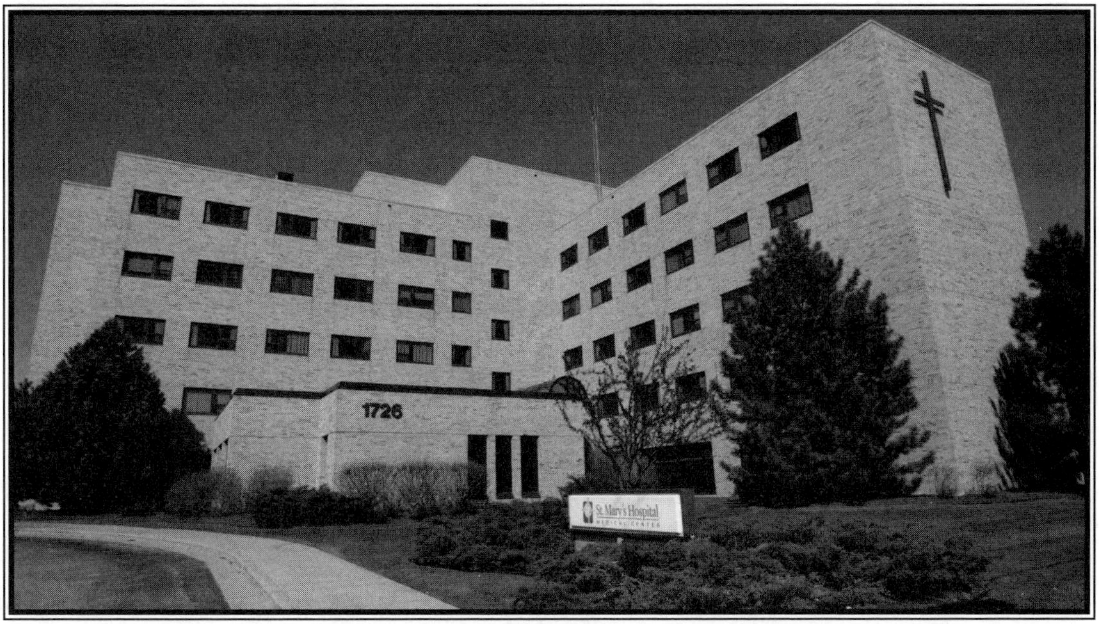

Photo courtesy of St. Mary's Hospital Medical Center

Bellin Hospital began planning for a new addition soon after their offer for St. Mary's was rejected. In August 1975 Dan Smith announced a proposed four story building on Van Buren Street. Four more stories could be added later. The structure was to house the cardiac surgery, cardiac catheterization lab, intensive care area, laboratory, x-ray, food service, and a conference room. Cost was projected as five million. The building would complete a square surrounding the courtyard used for parking. [21]

Several new medical services were introduced to the area in the 1970's. One of these was medical oncology. St. Vincent was interested in developing a regional cancer treatment center. They had established a radiotherapy unit and had radiation oncologists already in the hospital but wanted to expand their service with the addition of a medical oncology service. Dr. Stewart Adair, pediatrician, Dr. Robert Johnston, and Dr. Jim Lacey, internists, had been doing much of the cancer treatment although they did general medicine also. St. Vincent brought in Dr. Paul Koch who completed an oncology fellowship at Brown University Rhode Island Hospital. Dr. Koch opened an office July 1976 in St. Vincent Hospital. Within three years, Dr. Gerald Bayer arrived after a hematology fellowship at Case Western Reserve in Ohio to associate with Dr. Koch. The group continued to grow with the addition of Dr. Jim McGovern in 1985 after he completed his oncology training at Rhode Island Hospital.

Bellin Hospital established one of the first Hospice units in the state under Dr. Tom Leicht, an internist with the Beaumont Clinic. Dr. Leicht was very much concerned with the care of the dying and in conjunction with Dan Smith, Bellin's administrator, was instrumental in developing an in-patient unit. Dr. Leicht became the initial medical director of the Carl Kouba Hospice Unit, named after the late chairman of the hospital board. Over time the hospice concept evolved into a combined inpatient-outpatient service with minimal use of hospital beds.

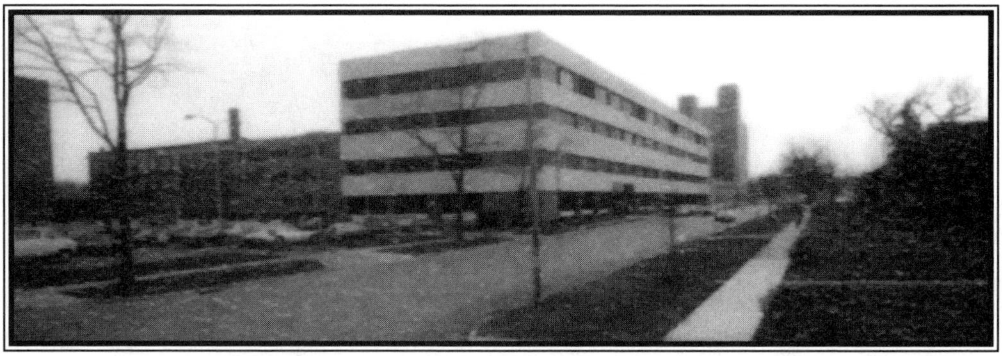

Photo courtesy of Bellin Health

By the beginning of the 1980's most of the medical subspecialties were represented in Brown County. The family practice residency graduates were also returning to Northeast Wisconsin. The absolute number of physicians arriving in Brown County was increasing and the role of each new doctor was better defined than in the previous decade.

The first doctor to do colonoscopies in Green Bay was Dr. Frank McCollough. He received his gastroenterlogy training at Ohio State University before joining the Deckner Clinic in 1973. Dr. McCullough decided to go back to Toledo, Ohio after ten years in Wisconsin. He became a faculty member of the Ohio State Medical School in Toledo and eventually rose to the position of dean of the school. Gastroenterology services were continued in Brown County by Dr. Len Wahl and Dr. Narayan Amarnani who both arrived in 1979.

One of the last subspecialties of internal medicine represented in Green Bay was infectious diseases. Dr. Dale Davis provided much needed expertise in the field diagnosis and treatment of infections. The old standard antibiotics were still used but were rapidly being replaced by new and more potent drugs needed to treat antibiotic resistant bacteria and newly recognized non-bacterial disease pathogens.

Plastic surgery is usually defined as cosmetic in nature. Dr. Hal Hoops was the pioneer in the area of plastic surgery. Mayo Clinic trained, he came to Green Bay in 1964. At the time, he was the only one in his specialty outside of Milwaukee and Madison. He brought in Dr. Ed Jacobs in 1970. In the first years, Dr. Hoops did a lot of emergency repair work and never had time to do extensive cosmetic surgery. Gradually, he and his partners were able to do more cosmetic surgery as a result of other surgical specialists and emergency physicians expanding their roles.

The older family practice physicians were doing less of the surgery and their places were taken by the physicians who arrived after 1960. The newly arrived surgeons were more extensively trained and contributed to a new era of more complex pre- and post-operative care. In addition to those already mentioned, Drs. Jim Curl, Jack Swelsted, and Thomas Geocaris were trained in general and vascular surgery. Dr. Robert Brault practiced thoracic and general surgery. Each had a busy practice and advanced the reputation of surgery in the area.

Notes to Chapter 11

1. *Press-Gazette*, July 1, 1970.
2. *Press-Gazette*, August 20, 1971.
3. *Press-Gazette*, October 4, 1970.
4. *Press-Gazette*, November 12, 1978.
5. Sehring, Dr. Fred. Report to the St. Vincent Executive Committee, April 21, 1981.
6. A Health Systems Plan for Northeastern Wisconsin 1978-83, published by the Northeastern Wisconsin Health Systems Agency, Inc. and funded by the Department of Health Education and Welfare through a Health Systems Agency Planning Grant, September 1, 1977.
7. Schlueter, Clyde F., President Employers Insurance of Wausau, *Doctors and Insurance*, a pamphlet prepared by the Company emphasizing the problems causing rising malpractice premiums and the cost to the patient, 1975.
8. *Press-Gazette*, March 27, 1974.
9. Dettmann, John E. MD *Wisconsin State Medical Journal* vol. 73, pg. 12 November 1974.
10. Johnston, Dr. Robert and Green, Dr. Jeremy, personal communication.
11. Brown County Medical Society Minutes April 12, 1973 and News Release.
12. *Press-Gazette*, April 27,1973.
13. ibid.
14. *Press-Gazette*, May 5, 1973 Supreme Court Decision, June 3, 1973, Appeals court decision.

15. ibid March 28, 1974.
16. ibid, December 8. 1973.
17. See note 15.
18. *Press-Gazette*, July 3, 1974.
19. ibid, March 3, 1978.
20. ibid, March 8, 1978.
21. ibid, August 5, 1975.

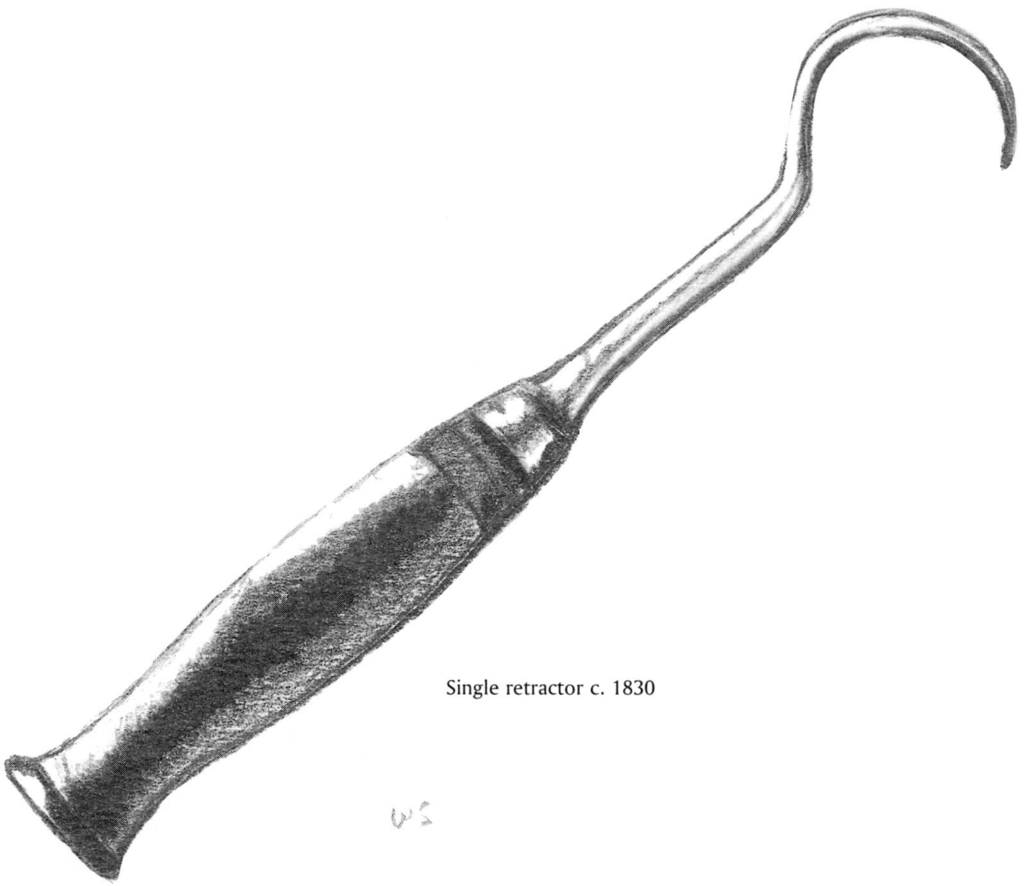

Single retractor c. 1830

Chapter 12

Physician-Hospital Groups

The last two decades of the twentieth century witnessed further transition in medical care from an individual doctor or small group to the much more complex multi-specialty clinic with hospital integration. Doctors' decision making came under increasing control of third party insurers and the patient-physician relationship became subject to the financial goals of the larger organization. The medical society, which had represented individual physicians, was no longer the consensus building or authoritative body. The hospital-clinic assumed more control of daily medical practice and economic issues confronting physicians. Competition for the health care dollar was between large hospital-physician groups and not between individual doctors. High profile advertising for the hospital-physician group appealed directly to the consumer. The individual physician had an increasingly difficult role to assume as patient advocate at the same time he or she was a member of a larger hospital-physician group, and unwillingly subject to the expanding array of "cost saving" measures promulgated by insurance companies and the various government agencies monitoring physicians.

The 1970's had seen a reversal in the ratio of family practice to specialty doctors in Green Bay. The number of specialists increased dramatically during this time. A few of the specialties were difficult to recruit to Brown County. The clinics often were unable to compete for the specialists because of the prevailing high salaries and the inability to ensure a competitive income for the initial years of practice. The hospitals were in a better financial position to recruit key specialists and give them a guaranteed salary and expenses, often including office space. After 1980, few physicians who desired to practice in Green Bay accepted the economic hazard of a solo office. There was much more to beginning a practice than putting the shingle out and waiting for the patients to come. Office rent and equipment were only a fraction of the cost. Medical school debts, malpractice premiums, computer billing systems, and additional employees with experience in the complexities of insurance were added cost considerations which the doctors of the post-WW II era did not have to face.

Radiologists, pathologists, and anesthesiologists were hospital based for decades. The emergency room physicians had office space within the hospital. These doctors were an integral part of the hospital function. Gradually, the hospitals began to hire other physicians who were not ordinarily considered hospital based. Bellin hired cardiologists to start their cardiology program. Oncology offices were established at St. Vincent to accommodate the oncologist. A cardiac surgeon was brought to Green Bay by Bellin Hospital. Physicians who had their own offices were beginning to be more concerned over the presumed unfair competitive advantage the hospital-based physician had obtained.

In a report prepared in 1977 for the Bellin hospital board by Dr. Richard Troup the issue of hospital employment of physicians was addressed, in reference to the hiring of a paid physician for hospice service. One anonymous comment expressed the concern of most doctors. “The fact remains, however, that they (hospital administration) are in many cases subsidizing services which are in direct competition with those of us who have come here on our own and invested our own borrowed money to establish medical care. I can not help but feel that this is only the beginning of hospital based employees and that while it will probably not occur during my professional career, that in years to come the hospital will employ more and more physicians for more and more services.” [1]

The report concluded that the physician community was opposed to employment of doctors by the hospital except in instances where the medical community felt that the service could not be provided by traditional fee for service practice. A temporary subsidy for a doctor in such cases was deemed reasonable but only for a limited time.

A similar report was prepared for the Brown County Medical Society in December 1979 by Dr. Joe Grace and Robert Schmidt, Jr. The report was a response to the preparation of office space in St. Vincent for Dr. Robert Gruesen, a neurosurgeon, and Dr. Fred Sehring, an obstetrician. The hospital had final plans drawn for the offices and was near the construction phase before the medical staff was able to convince the administration that providing office space in the hospital for physicians was contrary to the principles of the medical community. Fee for service, and independence from the hospital were the guiding principles of the position paper of the society. [2]

These reports were by physicians whose primary practice was at St. Vincent and Bellin and ignored the situation at St. Mary’s. Even before St. Mary’s was sold to the Third Order of St. Francis, the West Side Clinic was renting office space in the old nuns’ quarters of the hospital complex. Apparently, this was not a weakness in the argument against providing office space in the hospital for doctors. The oncologist at St. Vincent was also provided office space in the hospital, but his practice was thought to require the proximity of the hospital lab and x-ray to give better care. In general, contracts of physicians recruited and hired by the hospitals were for fee for service with a guaranteed base salary, but the location of offices within facilities owned by hospitals and the direct employment of physicians was proceeding despite the opposition of the majority of physicians.

In 1983 St. Vincent opened a rehabilitation facility on the second floor of the hospital. Dr. Lester Owens was recruited by the administration to be medical director. A graduate of the physical medicine training program at University of Missouri, he was the first physiatrist to come to Brown County. Previously, stroke victims and other neurologic problems requiring prolonged rehabilitation were treated at home, nursing homes, or the Curative Workshop by physical therapists under orders written by the attending physician. The Curative Workshop had for years provided therapy for the disabled and had been successful in building a respected program for the community. There was concern initially that the two programs would be competitive, but they actually became complementary.

Dr. Owens had an office and practice located in St. Vincent and although he was employed under contract with the hospital as medical director, his income was derived mostly from fee for service. The rehabilitation department was widely promoted by the hospital and two more physiatrists, Dr. Brock Robinson and Dr. Karen Heida soon arrived.

The number of women physicians has dramatically increased since 1980. From 1940 until 1975 when Dr. Karen Camilli joined the Beaumont Clinic pediatric staff, only a few women started practice in the county. None stayed very long. There were no women physicians in the 1969 photograph of the 116 members of the Brown County Medical Society. Dr. Kathleen Barkow, also a pediatrician, 1980; Dr. Sally Schlise, radiation oncologist, 1981; Patricia Blohowiak, family practice, 1982; began a gradual but steady increase in women engaged in medical care in Brown County. Dr. Colleen Corbett and Dr. Pam Dobson both ophthalmologists and Dr. Gayle Kasdorf, endocrinologist soon followed. By 2000, women were represented in most of the specialties including general surgery. Despite the greater numbers of women, positions of authority were still dominated by men. A reduction in nights and weekends on call, ease of referral to other specialists, full time emergency doctors, and more recently, the hospitalist programs have softened the realities of private practice in Brown County. The twenty-four hour work day, seven days a week of the past has been replaced by more reasonable hours. This is understandably more conducive to improved family life for both male and female physicians.

The Hospital board of directors and administrators had always listened to the professional opinions of physicians since the first hospital was opened in Brown County. The decisions of the hospital board, however, did not always please the medical community. The incumbent president of the medical staff was first represented on the board at Bellin in the early 1980's. Although Dr. Bellin had been president of the Bellin board earlier, the hospital board had been composed of Methodist pastors for many years and more recently businessmen from the community. In a departure from the past, the Sisters of the Third Order appointed Dr. Jack Killins as a voting member of the board in 1983 and for the first time included the administrator, Joe Neidenbach, and representatives of the community on the board. Both governing bodies apparently desired a physician with voting privileges to represent the doctors utilizing the facility. The physicians on the boards were respected by their peers and influential in the medical community but were out- numbered by community businessmen in the case of the Bellin Board and at St. Vincent by the Sisters of the Third Order of St. Francis.

The Medical Society influence in hospital decision making or in selecting physicians needed in the County was rapidly waning in the 1980's. One physician who remained active in the state society was Dr. Roger VON Heimburg. A graduate of Johns Hopkins, University of Minnesota-Rochester Medical School, the general surgery residency at the Mayo Clinic, and a member of the Webster Clinic, Roger was very active at the state level. After serving on the board of directors for ten years, he was elected president of the Wisconsin State Medical Society in 1990. Dr. VON Heimburg expressed his concern over the evolving relationship between patient and physician brought on by the increasing business mentality of medical care. "Government regulators, insurance companies, utilization review corporations, and the bottom liner at hospitals and clinics have twisted a warm, caring encounter into a cold lifeless business transaction. They reduce the art of healing to an act of selling." 3

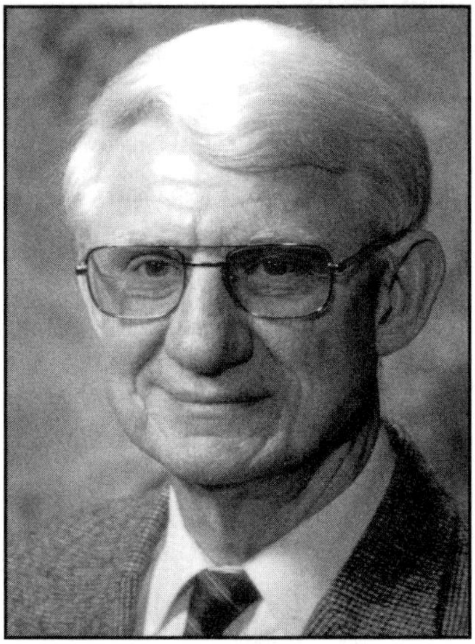

Dr. Roger VON Heimburg
1931 - 1999
Photo courtesy of
St. Vincent Hospital

A number of factors led to the greater influence of national medical organizations over the local medical community. The greater number of specialists and the peculiar concerns of each specialty led to a greater reliance on the specialty society for educational and economic information. Dr. Dan Shea had been involved with the American Academy of Pediatrics as a member of the board of directors because of his work on the national committee on ambulatory medicine. In 1990 he was elected vice-president of the American Academy of Pediatrics and a year later assumed the presidency of the organization. He was deeply involved in promoting practice guidelines, rewriting government vaccine pamphlets for patients, and enhancing the Academy membership. 4

Academic medicine in the form of basic research or clinical studies and the teaching of medical students, interns, and residents never received a high priority in Brown County. St. Mary's Hospital had abandoned the internship program in the late 1920's. The Green Bay Academy of Medicine had excellent goals but ceased to exist after WWII. The hospital staff organization required review of mortalities and case discussions but did not go further in promoting clinical research. Dr. Herb Sandmire organized a preceptorship for University of Wisconsin Medical School students in 1966 which lasted twenty years. He also was instrumental in developing a two-month residency program in obstetrics for family practice in 1980. In addition to his teaching responsibility, Dr. Sandmire published clinical research studies on controversial obstetrical issues including cesarean section birth rates. As a medical community, Brown County was not widely recognized in the state for research and teaching.

All three hospitals were accredited by the American Medical Association Council on Education to present educational programs. A complete residency program in family practice or other medical disciplines was never seriously contemplated. Other cities in Wisconsin with lesser referral areas developed close medical school ties and residency programs. Although pursuit of a medical school and post-graduate training were suggested at one time or another, cost and lack of interest dampened the enthusiasm. Today, many of the individual physicians and hospital departments maintain ties with teaching institutions but obstetrics is the only post-graduate teaching program.

The most significant concern of the medical community in the 1980's was the possible intrusion of an outside medical-hospital-insurance group that would disrupt the established physician- patient base. The rising cost of medical care was a force in the search for solutions. Nationwide, the emergence of HMO's (health maintenance organizations) PPO's (preferred provider organizations), and PHO's (physician-hospital organizations) were finding acceptance with the insurance industry, government, and in some areas, the patients. An outside organization could sell an insurance plan in the county which would exclude local physicians from their rolls and control patient referrals. Savings could result from efficiencies of a large group. The end result being a reduction in income for the small clinic or independent doctor.

Brown County physicians were also concerned about the high cost of health care. In 1978 and 1979, Dr. Jeremy Green led the medical society in a campaign to lower costs. More ambulatory care, fewer hospitalizations for laboratory or x-ray procedures, and elimination of the annual physical examination for healthy young people were ways in which physicians could reduce costs. [5] Keeping the cost of medical care in Brown County lower than the national average probably was a factor in excluding outside managed care plans.

The nation's medical schools responded to the relative lack of family doctors and instituted a three-year residency program in family practice with its own specialty board. The number of medical school graduates entering family practice residencies increased and resulted in the growing presence of the family doctor in the community. The smaller communities surrounding Green Bay had experienced a loss of their family doctors after WWII and now were beginning to see a return of the family practitioner to the outlying areas. In the most part they would be supported and affiliated with one of the larger organizations based in Green Bay.

In 1994 Bellin Hospital bought the Denmark Clinic practice from Dr. Hering and Kulkoski. That started a movement that rapidly attracted other family practice physicians to the Bellin Medical Group. Dr. Jim Jerzak and William Reynders, Ashwaubenon; Julio Artega, Brillion; Dr. Peri Aldrich, Pulaski; Dr. Mark Weise, Algoma; Drs. Chester Crawford and Wesley McNeal, Green Bay; Dr. Tom Zenner, Kewaunee; James Wallace, Peshtigo; and Dr. Vernette Carlson, Daggett, Michigan all became Bellin employees and sold their medical practices to Bellin. Because of more adequate funding and expertise in recruiting, the hospital was successful in hiring new physicians for these practices. In addition, the hospital employed the office staff and relieved the doctors of much of the business aspect of the practice. What began as a single office buyout soon became a network of primary care physicians in Northeast Wisconsin stretching from Brillion in the south to Marinette in the north and Bonduel in the west to Kewaunee on the lake shore. Obviously, physician referrals would more likely be to Bellin Hospital and justify the expense for the Hospital Corporation. New physicians were initially paid a guaranteed salary and then usually had a fee for service contract. Bellin chose not to employ specialists.

St. Vincent Hospital had attempted to organize an outpatient surgery center with a group of specialists who were interested. The cost of procedures done in the hospital far exceeded the cost of the same procedure done at an in-hospital operating room (OR). The overhead expense for twenty-four hour, seven day a week OR could not compete with an outpatient facility with no night or weekend personnel. The hospital and specialists did not follow through and the project was eventually dropped.

The Green Bay Eye Clinic was instrumental in developing an independent outpatient surgery center. Bay Care, which included the Eye Clinic and other surgical specialists, was organized in 1994. They opened a surgery center on the West side of Green Bay in 1995. The members of Bay Care realized any profits derived from the outpatient OR fee as well as their professional fee. The immediate impact of this on the hospitals was a reduction of income from the procedures now being performed in the outpatient surgery center by the ophthalmologists and other specialists. The response from Bellin and St. Vincent was to aggressively lower their outpatient surgery costs and attempt to retain as much of the surgery as possible. In effect the community benefited, at least temporarily, from the price reductions

Dr. Henry Majeski and Dr. Henry Rahr, family practice doctors, were for many years the Luxemburg Clinic. They approached St. Vincent Hospital to buy their practice about the same time Bellin was buying their first primary care practices. Joe Neidenbach, administrator and the board agreed to purchase the practice although their intent was not to own private offices. St. Vincent instead actively pursued the Webster Clinic and Beaumont Clinic physicians in 1995. Both Clinics had been talking about a merger. It was not long before the West Side Clinic, located near St. Mary's Hospital began talks with the two East side Clinics. The result of negotiations was the formation of Prevea Clinic, a fifty-fifty joint venture between St. Vincent and St. Mary's and the three multispecialty clinics. The Hospitals brought the financial resources for expansion of the group to Prevea and the Clinic brought patients to the hospitals. Interestingly, Green Bay is the only area served by the Third Order of St. Francis that has a hospital-clinic joint venture. [6]

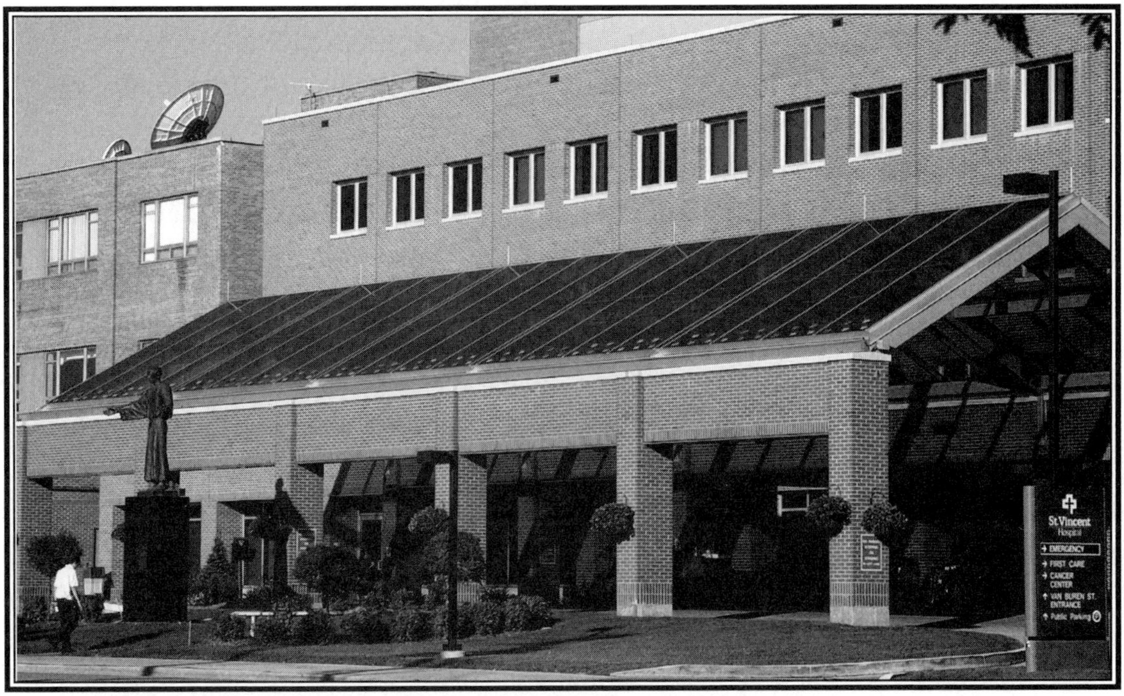

Photo courtesy of St. Vincent Hospital

While Bellin and St. Vincent-St. Mary's were trying to protect their market share by forming associations with physicians in the area, a new player in the grand game of health care monopoly appeared on the scene. Aurora, centered in Milwaukee with clinics and hospitals from Kenosha to Manitowoc, purchased the Deckner Clinic and Green Bay Clinic in 1994. Soon Dr. Don Sipes, Ed Vogel, and Richard Shaffer, obstetricians joined. Within a brief period Aurora had established clinics in De Pere, Allouez, Algoma, Sturgeon Bay, Marinette, and Peshtigo. Dr. Tom Kohler, an internist with the former Deckner Clinic, who had earned a MBA degree from University of Wisconsin became president of the Northern Region of Aurora. By 1996 all of Northeast Wisconsin was divided into three separate health provider entities. This left Bay Care, the group of surgical specialists and emergency doctors looking for an association. There were a few other independent specialists not affiliated with any of the three groups. These included neurologists, nephrologists, infectious disease specialists, endocrinologists, and orthopedists.

The Bay Care group, comprised of the emergency doctors, eye, ear, nose and throat doctors, general surgeons, orthopedists, and urologists first tried to reach an agreement with Prevea and then Bellin Hospital before associating with Aurora and forming a forty: sixty financial partnership which merged the outpatient surgery centers and a projected new hospital into a for-profit organization named Bay Care Aurora Medical Center to be located just East of Highway 43 and Mason Street.

A significant addition and remodeling took place in 1999-2000 at St. Vincent. New office space for an expanded oncology service and more space for the radiology department was built. Administrative staff and much needed meeting rooms occupied the third and fourth floors of the new building. Ironically, the expanded emergency room was manned by a new group of emergency doctors and the Bay Care doctors that helped plan the facility were now working for Aurora.

Another important project was the construction and equipping of a cardiac catheterization lab at St. Mary's Hospital. Dr. Peter Fergus, who once had been associated with Dr. Palay and Anthony at Bellin, lobbied successfully for a cardiac procedure room at St. Mary's. All open heart surgery was still done at Bellin. This was the first stone cast at Bellin's monopoly on heart catheterization in Brown County, but Bay Care Aurora Medical Center was expected to open their own cardiac center in the new hospital.

Psychiatry as a medical specialty was introduced to Brown County in the 1940's. Treatment of the mentally ill, although important in overall patient care, is not usually considered a high revenue source in comparison to surgery. The history of psychiatry in Brown County is of interest because of the financial forces which eventually determined the major delivery system. This will be discussed in the next chapter.

Notes to Chapter 12

1. Report to the Bellin Hospital board of directors from a survey of the medical staff, Dr. Richard Troup. This survey was in reaction to the hospice program and the hiring of a medical director by the hospital.
2. Report to Brown County Medical Society, Guidelines and Principles for Physician Recruitment and Hospital Relationship, Prepared by Dr. Joe Grace, Dr. Charles Smith, and Dr. Robert Kaftan. Presented at December 4, 1979. The report was also presented to the hospital administrators and discussed at St. Vincent Medical staff meetings.
3. VON Heimburg, Dr. Roger, presidential address to Wisconsin State Medical Society, *Wisconsin State Medical Journal* vol. 89, July 1990.
4. Shea, Dr. Dan, personal communication.
5. *Press-Gazette*, May 6, 1978. written by Sarah Watke who reported frequently on medical topics for the *Press-Gazette* for several years.
6. Neidenbach, Joe, Administrator St. Vincent Hospital, 1982-present, personal communication.

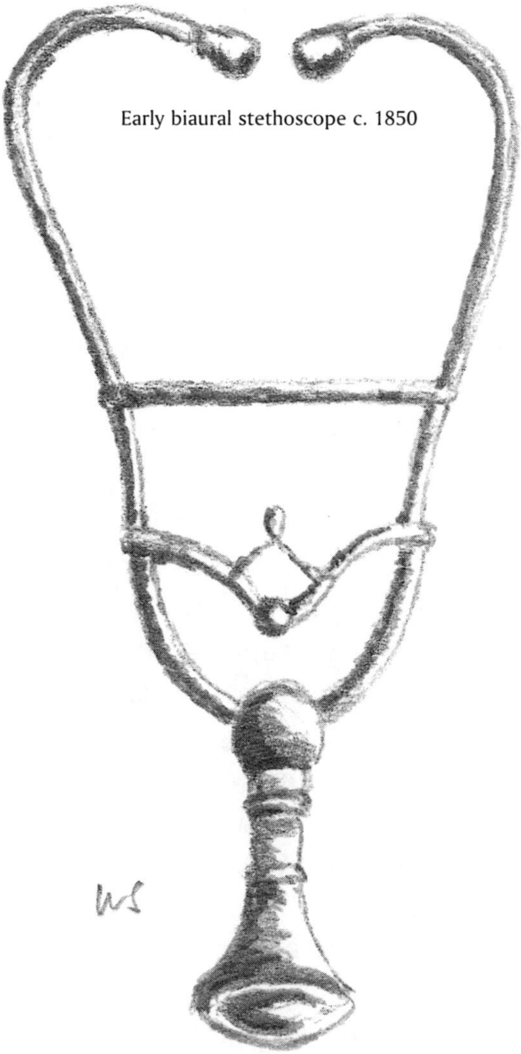

Early biaural stethoscope c. 1850

Chapter 13
Psychiatry

Psychiatry as a specialty of medicine was introduced to Brown County in the early 1940's. The understanding and definition of mental illness was evolving into a systematic classification based upon signs and symptoms of a disease. Prior to this time patients were separated from society and treatment was aimed more at controlling symptoms than cure. The concept of permanently confining the insane to an institution without hope of release was being challenged. Phenobarbital, bromides, chloral hydrate, opium, and hot baths were in use to control behavior. Electroconvulsive and insulin shock therapy were important therapeutic modalities. Psychiatry was changing from the Freudian psychoanalytic focus to a psychobiologic and psychodynamic approach to treatment. Training programs for psychiatry included the study of psychopathology, nervous system disorders, psychology, and basic psychiatric science. The intent was to provide doctors who were better qualified to treat disease rather than isolate children and adults with mental illness. The American Board of Psychiatry and Neurology set standards for residencies and began certifying psychiatrists in 1934.

Recognizing the importance of treating abnormal behavior and mental illness, Brown County hired the first psychiatrist in the area. Dr. Elizabeth Kane was employed at the Brown County Guidance Center beginning in 1940. She continued in that position until 1955 although she began a part-time private practice in 1946. Dr. Kane was born in Kane, Pennsylvania, the granddaughter of a pioneering woman physician of the same name. The younger Dr. Kane had extensive training for seven years before confining her practice to psychiatry. A graduate of Loyola Medical School in Chicago, she completed a general internship in LaCrosse, Wisconsin and then spent a year in Rawalpindi, India as a missionary doctor before embarking on her psychiatric study. Her itinerary took her to Jersey City, Boston Psychopathic, Milwaukee and finally a year at Johns Hopkins Hospitals. [1] The primary focus of her study was psychiatric-based child guidance. Much like her grandmother who began the first hospital in Kane, Pennsylvania in 1873, Dr. Elizabeth Kane pioneered psychiatry in Brown County. Bringing a new discipline to the area in addition to being accepted as a female physician in a male-dominated profession was a noteworthy achievement.

The first psychiatrist to venture an adult private practice in Green Bay was Dr. Charles Wunsch. He was certified by the American Board of Psychiatry and Neurology after a three year residency in neuropsychiatry at St. Joseph's Retreat Hospital in Detroit. Following two years in the Air Force, Dr. Wunsch entered the private practice of psychiatry in 1953 with an office in the Bellin Building.

Treatment or more realistically, isolation, of the mental cases, derelicts, disabled vagrants, and alcoholics had been at the Brown County Home beginning in 1858. The Home was built on Bay Settlement Road on one hundred twelve acres of farmland. Thirty-nine individuals including two families with seven children each were the first "patients." Dr. David Ward, the first civilian physician in Brown County was appointed physician in charge. The facility was renamed the Brown County Insane Asylum in 1881 and for the first time the insane were housed in a separate building. General physicians were appointed to care for patients although there were few medications available to treat the underlying psychiatric and medical conditions. In addition to housing for the patients and the caretaker, an institutional farm supplied much of the produce for the inmates and provided cash for care of the patients. A dairy herd and later an apple orchard were maintained by the patients. A new facility for two hundred patients costing $300,000 was eventually built at the same site in 1935 and the name changed to the Brown County Hospital in 1948. Patients with more acute and severe mental illness were eligible to be sent to the State Mental Hospital. Until 1962, most of the patients housed at Brown County Hospital were chronically ill. In 1968, a new seventy-two bed psychiatric building was added to the complex and a children's unit opened. [2]

The acceptance of mental illness as a disease, the lack of a private facility for patients, and the more universal payment of hospital costs by insurance companies were factors which influenced St. Vincent Hospital to open a psychiatric unit in the new ten-story patient wing in 1957. Dr. Wunsch assisted the Sisters of the Third Order of St. Francis in developing the new service for the community. The second floor of the hospital had a locked unit and accepted acutely disturbed psychiatric patients. The presence of trained psychiatrists and the introduction of effective drug therapy also may have prompted the decision to provide a hospital-based treatment facility. Medications to control psychotic behavior such as the phenothiazines (Thorazine) were changing the care of acutely ill patients. This was the beginning of the pharmacological era of psychiatry. Dr. Bernard Kalina, trained at the University of Iowa psychiatric program, was temporarily associated with Dr. Wunsch. Soon Dr. James Caffrey, Dr. John Gehring, Dr. David Donarski, and Clarence Rothe, all fully trained psychiatrists, became partners in Psychiatric Services with offices in the Bellin Building. [3] Later they were joined by Dr. Harold Reinhart who had trained at Warren State Hospital in Pennsylvania.

Dr. Caffrey, a Marquette Medical School graduate, completed his specialty training at the Warren, Pennsylvania State Hospital and began his psychiatric practice about 1959. Dr. John Gehring also received his MD from Marquette but had his psychiatric training at the Cherokee, Iowa Mental Institute. Dr. Gehring arrived in Green Bay in 1963. Three years latter, Dr. David Donarski became the fourth member of the group. A native of Green Bay, educated at Marquette Medical School and the Warren State Hospital in Pennsylvania, he further enhanced the group's psychiatric domain which included most of northeast Wisconsin. Shortly thereafter Dr. Clarence Rothe also joined the Wunsch group from the psychiatric residency at Warren State Hospital. Dr. Rothe had been in general practice in Green Bay for several years before his specialty training.

Brown County Hospital had started admitting acute mentally ill patients in 1962. Most private pay or insured patients, however, were still hospitalized at St. Vincent Hospital. Brown County Hospital psychiatrists were involved in treatment of mental illness and a general physician was responsible for medical care. Dr. Caffrey and Dr. Gehring worked part time at the Mental Health Center and were succeeded by Dr. Eleanor Kuehn, a graduate of Marquette Medical School and the Wood Veterans Hospital Psychiatry program. She was hired as a full time psychiatrist by Brown County Hospital in 1969. Dr. Michael O'Neil became Medical Director of the renamed Brown County Mental Health Center in 1975.

Dr. Edward Orman and Dr. Leo Grieben started an adult psychiatric unit in 1978 and later an adolescent and children's ward at Bellin Hospital. Perceived administrative interference in patient care at St. Vincent Hospital prompted the two psychiatrists to respond to a proposal to initiate a psychiatric unit at Bellin Hospital. The new service was encouraged by Dan Smith, administrator of Bellin. The psychiatric program, including an alcohol detoxification unit for in-patients was successful and eventually encompassed a total of forty-two beds. The twelve-bed adolescent unit was established in 1985 and a children's treatment program developed in 1988. [4]

A graduate of University of Wisconsin Medical School and the psychiatric residency program, Dr. Orman also had a two-year residency in child psychiatry at the same institution. Dr. Orman had practiced adult and child psychiatry for six years in La Crosse prior to coming to Green Bay in late 1974.

A native of Argentina, Dr. Leo Grieben finished a psychiatry residency at the University of Minnesota before starting practice in Eau Claire, Wisconsin. In 1977, he associated with Dr. Orman, forming a second psychiatric group practice in the area. They would be joined by Drs. Norma Cruz and John Edrozo to form Bay Psychiatric. Psychiatric units were now established at St. Vincent, Bellin, and Brown County

Mental Health Center. Psychiatry had assumed a more traditional role in main-stream medical practice and was economically viable for the institutions, although Brown County Hospital was partially supported by tax dollars. Those patients who were indigent or had no insurance were usually treated at Brown County.

Psychiatric Institutes of America (PIA), a national for-profit hospital chain, entered the Green Bay market at a time when insurance companies were providing more coverage for psychiatric illnesses. A facility designed as a free standing psychiatric hospital was built in 1989 by PIA and the parent company, National Medical Enterprises, on St. Josephs Avenue in Allouez. It was named Fox Valley Hospital (FVH), presumably to attract patients from south of Green Bay. FVH became the fifty-sixth hospital in twenty-eight states owned by PIA. Dr. Michael O'Neil accepted the post of medical director. A graduate of Notre Dame and the University of Chicago Pritzker School of Medicine, Dr. O'Neil earned his board certification in Psychiatry after finishing a residency at University of Wisconsin. Dr. Howard W. Davis was appointed medical director for children and adolescent services. Dr. Davis had his education at Indiana University Medical School and a residency in adult psychiatry followed by a two-year program in child psychiatry at the same institution. He was board certified in both child and adult psychiatry. Prior to his appointment at FVH he had been clinical director at Brown County Mental Health Center 1982-1986 and in private practice. Dr. Edward Johnson was to head the chemical dependency program. Dr. Johnson's psychiatry training was at Medical College of Wisconsin and the affiliated hospitals. He also was clinical director of the Brown County Mental Health Center 1978-1982. [5]

The nine million dollar Fox Valley Hospital was designed to have a potential of eighty in-patient beds and provide outpatient services. A full range of psychiatric care was offered for adults, adolescents, and children. Office space for the psychiatrists and therapists was included in the well-equipped structure. The philosophy of Fox Valley Hospital was "to return people as quickly as possible to a normal life in the community, home, and school. Through intensive structured therapy programs involving individual, group, family, school and expressive activities, patients are encouraged to take on new skills for coping with the pressures and problems of daily living." [6]

Reacting to the announced opening of Fox Valley hospital and its own high in-patient census, Bellin decided to build a modern facility devoted to psychiatry. St. Vincent Hospital's patient census was declining and the psychiatric community supported Bellin's building proposal. Events surrounding hospital care of patients began to take place rapidly. Bellin's psychiatric hospital was in the process of being built when Fox Valley opened for business in June 1989. On May 1, 1990, St. Vincent closed the psychiatric floor and ended thirty-two years of hospital in-patient mental illness care. The reasons were decreasing census, increasing competition for patients, and the higher ratio of non-paying patients being referred to the hospital. One month after St. Vincent closed, Bellin opened the new Psychiatric Center on Webster Avenue directly across from the main hospital. For almost a year there were four psychiatric facilities operating in Brown County.

Fox Valley Psychiatric Hospital was the first for-profit hospital in the area other than the physician operated homes prior to the founding of St. Vincent Hospital. The Fox Valley Hospital and physician employees were managed by a local administration and an absentee corporate board which answered to the owners, Psychiatric Institutes of America. Insurance payments for mental illness hospitalization and psychiatric care were quite favorable at the time. Hospital stays were often prolonged and beds were easily filled with patients. A profit was almost assured if claims to the insurance company were properly filed. Initially, the hospital did well with a high census and community support thanks in part to the aggressive publicity campaign. Changes in insurance reimbursement and shortening hospital stays began to impact the economics of the facility. Charges of unethical practices by Psychiatric Institues of America surfaced in the media initially from other hospitals in the chain and later in Green Bay. It was alleged that criteria for admission were sometimes marginal and that as soon as the patient's insurance benefit was used up the patient was discharged regardless of the status of recovery from illness. Dr. O'Neil, who resigned his position before the hospital closed, was increasingly aware of the higher costs of care at FVH and the subtle pressure of administration to prolong hospital stay and increase the census. Apparently, the profit motive was deemed more important than the original mission outlined in the philosophy. Careful review of patient records did not reveal any physician deception. [7]

Fox Valley Hospital opened June 10, 1989 with a day long celebration which featured a national television actor, a clown, and puppets. It closed in the fall of 1993 with much less orchestrated publicity. The hospital had been offered for sale in October 1992 but had not found a buyer. The in-patient census gradually declined until closure. The vacant building was a reminder of a failed venture and of the possible purchase by another psychiatric for-profit company. PIA was forced out of existence and National Medical Enterprises was in need of cash.

Meanwhile, Bellin Hospital was in need of more room for the Nursing School, the hospital gastrointestinal lab, and the new Bellin Medical Group of family practitioners. Purchasing the vacant Fox Valley Hospital for their psychiatric patients would prevent another psychiatric entity from coming to Green Bay, provide room for the needed expansion, and the price was exceptionally favorable. On June 30, 1994 Bellin purchased the Fox Valley Hospital for $980,000 and moved the Bellin Psychiatric Center to the facility on St. Joseph's Street. The hospital had been built for a cost of eight and one-half million dollars. The purchase price included all the furnishings and equipment in the building. Only the computer systems were removed. After the move, four psychiatric centers had been reduced to two in-patient facilities within a five year span. [8]

Over the next six years the treatment of mental illness became even more outpatient oriented and hospital stays were significantly reduced largely due to more effective drug therapy. The number of fully trained psychiatrists in 1994 totaled fifteen, divided into two groups, Bay Psychiatric Services (a section of Bellin Medical Group) and Riverside Psychiatric. Only a few psychiatrists were independent. Five of the doctors were actively engaged in adolescent and child psychology. In addition, Brown County Hospital employed at least one full time psychiatrist. Prominent among the more recent arrivals were Drs. Peter Fischer, Neil Fullan, Chris Larson, Koti Mannen, Brad Lyles, George Soncrant, John Stamm, Jon Thomas, and Edwin Watts. Brown County was the only center for psychiatric services for a large region of northeastern Wisconsin. Changes in public awareness and policy toward mental illness, insurance benefit mandates, supportive public and private hospital administrators, and energetic physicians combined to ensure a highly successful psychiatric service in the area.

Notes to Chapter 13

1. Application for membership for the Brown County Medical Society, Feb 15, 1946, Elizabeth D. Kane MD. Brown County Medical Society Historical file.
2. History of Brown County Mental Health Center, 1858-1983, 125 Years of Service, Brown County Library Historical Section, 1983.
3. Donarski, David, personal communication.
4. Orman, Edward, personal communication.
5. *Green Bay Press-Gazette*, June 4, 1989.
6. ibid., June 12, 1989.
7. O'Neil, Michael, personal communication.
8. Fry, Robert, personal communication. Bob Fry was president of Bellin Psychiatric Center at its inception and moved the Center to the Fox Valley facility when Bellin purchased the building on St. Joseph's Street.

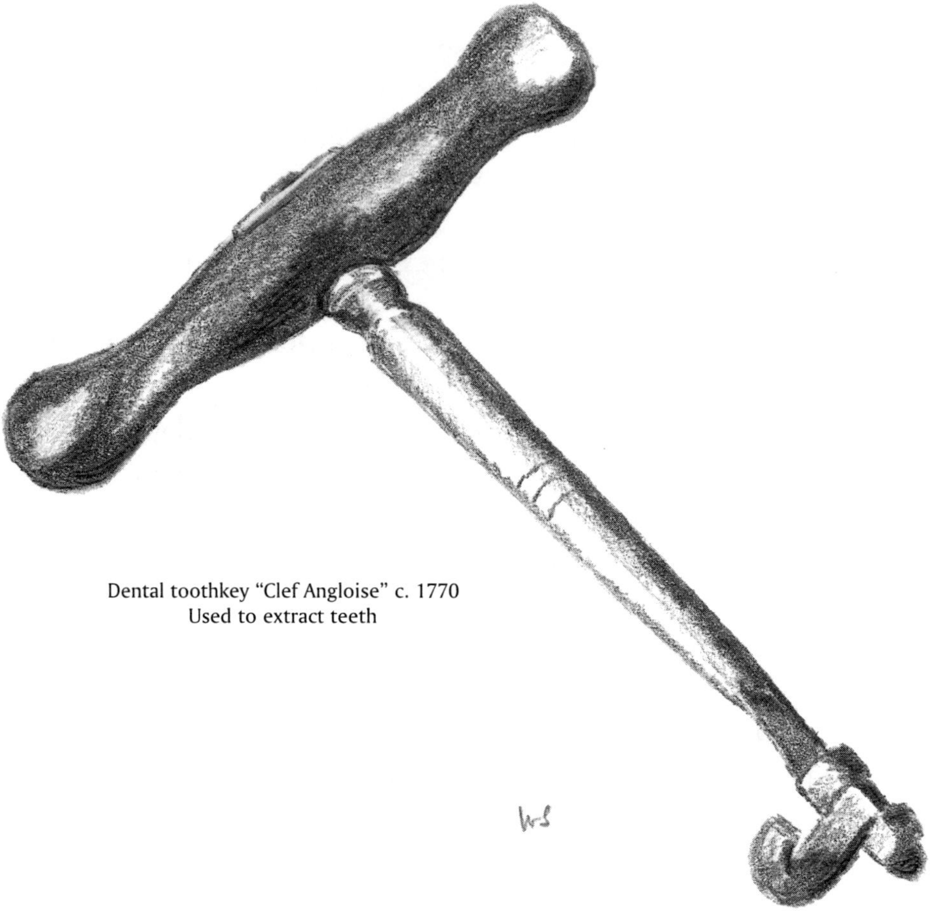

Dental toothkey "Clef Angloise" c. 1770
Used to extract teeth

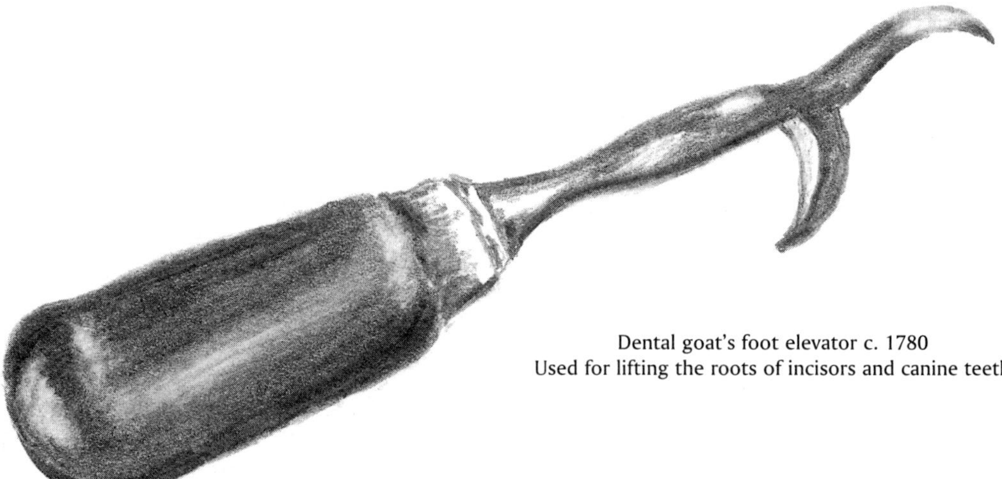

Dental goat's foot elevator c. 1780
Used for lifting the roots of incisors and canine teeth

Chapter 14

Patient-Physician Relationship

The days of the individual or the personality-based practice of medicine have gone and will not likely ever return to Brown County. Technologic and market driven forces positioned the individual physician in a multispecialty group practice for purpose of economy and efficiency at the same time attempting to fulfill the basic principles of caring for the sick with compassion in the traditional patient-physician relationship.

Physicians, except for a few independents, were separated into three distinct groups, Prevea, Bellin Medical Group, and Bay Care-Aurora Medical Group. Each had its primary base or in the case of the latter, the Bay Care Aurora Medical Center Hospital was to be occupied in 2001. Bellin was planning an addition to the Van Buren building in 2001-2002 and replacing the old hospital, built in 1915-25, the next year. St. Vincent had just completed an expansion of the Emergency Center and a new administrative area. St. Mary's was not planning any major changes. Both Bay Care Aurora and Prevea had plans for new physician clinic buildings within Brown County.

Physicians were either paid a salary, had a guaranteed minimum income with a production incentive, or were in some cases paid entirely by fee for service. All three physician hospital groups were aggressively recruiting new physicians in an attempt to bring both primary care and a full complement of specialists to the area. The competition for doctors gave the incoming physician a comfortable income in addition to an office and the equipment necessary for his or her specialty. The doctor did not have to endure the hard times of physicians of the previous generations whose first few years in practice were often a struggle to survive.

Managed care in the form of HMO's and PPO's competed with indemnity insurance for patients. Medicine had taken on a business model with each group having a structure enabling the entity to compete for the health care dollar. Prevea Clinic established the Prevea Health Plan and a HMO. Bellin Medical Group participated in Touchpoint, a PPO and HMO based in the Fox Valley although Bellin Medical and Prevea both welcomed indemnity insurance patients. Bay Care and the Aurora Medical Group relied on the indemnity insurance sector for their market share after Aurora opted out of Touchpoint. Independent physicians who wanted to treat patients in the HMO and PPO plans had to sign contracts to provide services at discounts from their usual fees or the patients had to pay out of pocket for services. Patients consulting independent doctors who did not subscribe to the managed care plans used their indemnity insurance or those without insurance paid fees themselves. All groups participated in Medicare and Medicaid although some independent physicians limited their Medicaid patients.

One of the controversies surrounding the managed care plans was the concept of the gatekeeper. Rising costs in medical care were thought to be at least partially due to the higher cost of specialty services and in rare cases inappropriate use of procedures and care provided by specialists. Traditionally, patients could seek out the specialist on their own and by-pass the primary care doctor. The gatekeeper concept was an attempt to limit specialty care cost by requiring the patient to have a referral by the primary care physician (gatekeeper) or the plan would not pay for the service. In Brown County, referral to specialists by the primary care doctor was generally very appropriate. Sanctions or financial penalties for referring to specialties were not a factor in the clinics although the implied threat of financial loss to the provider was always present. The cost of medical services was slowed by the efficiencies of managed care plans but by 1999 costs were again rising at an alarming rate in Brown County.

Medical costs have been a concern for over thirty years. One of the traditions that has disappeared with time was the waiving of fees by physicians for patients deemed unable to pay for needed services. It was the treating physician's choice not to charge a patient as has been noted in an earlier chapter. Now the government has partially assumed that role by providing insurance payment for the poor or those who qualify for medical assistance. Medicare insurance provides partial payment for care of the elderly. Those who qualify by income level may receive Medicaid. Unfortunately, not all the poor are covered by government insurance and counties or cities often will contribute to care. In Brown County, the Green Bay Free Clinic also is available for those who cannot afford insurance. Few physicians, currently, do not submit a charge for service. Courtesy for medical personnel has been discouraged. The federal government has gone further. A physician may be charged with fraud if the co-payment is waived for a Medicare patient. The billing department of the climic corporation has the responsibility to collect fees and may forfeit fees in some instances without physician direction. The hospitals and clinics do write off charges that are deemed uncollectable. The concept of free care for the poor as an intregal part of the patient-physician relationship survives only in voluntary work outside the multispecialty group.

The most significant changes in medicine since the first doctors came to the shores of the Fox River are found not only in the tremendous advances in knowledge and the technologies created. The patient-physician relationship has been altered. No longer does the patient have an unwritten bond exclusively with his physician. The large group to which the physician belongs and the insurance carrier for the patient may hover over the medical decisions the doctor and patient make. Patients have more information and a larger role in decisions. The patient as a consumer of health care may dictate which provider will deliver a service within the bounds of a managed care contract. Conflicts between the consumer, provider, and the insurance company may be decided by a neutral mediator. In the past, the family doctor made the decisions. That trust has been dissected into a weakened relationship.

One result of the changing relationship may be the gradual and significant growth of non-traditional medicine in Brown County. The growth of the "natural medicine" industry and the increasing dependence of patients on practitioners of acupuncture, chiropractic, massage, and other healing modalities is part of the late twentieth century evolution of medical care. Traditional medicine has always been suspect because of ever-changing dogma and the acceptance of many unproved theories. The high cost of diagnosis, surgical treatment, and pharmacological therapy; presumed profit motive of doctors, and the complex system of corporate medicine may have enhanced the reliance on the non-traditional forms of care. Renewed interest in the old ways suggests the new is not the final answer to health care. The advertising of non-traditional modalities of care and herbal medications has similarities to the mid-nineteen century reaction to medical practices of the period.

As with many consumer-oriented businesses advertising has become important in gaining market share and influencing patient decisions. The American Medical Association had for many years discouraged direct advertising of physician services and restricted the ads to name, location and office hours. Physicians in Green Bay assiduously adhered to that policy until the 1980's. In the late 1960's, one MD was severely criticized for having his name in bold print in the physician section of the local phone book. Today, radio, newspaper, and television are replete with direct patient appeals to utilize services that are sometimes promoted as superior to competitors or at least of necessity to the individual. Many ads are only marginally important to the health of the patient and are clearly a means of increasing income for the doctor. For example, laser technology has fostered an advertising explosion for ophthalmologic procedures.

Further diminishing the doctor-patient relationship is the role the employer has in deciding which insurance product the employees may accept as part of a benefit package. Changing plans often means the patient loses his or her physician to the economics of business. On the other side, physicians may change groups or be fired from their clinic and the patient has to shop for a new doctor, all of which leads to a tenuous doctor-patient relationship.

Another result of the segregation of physicians into the three groups in Brown County is the change in cohesiveness of the entire medical community. Physicians are less likely to socialize and confer between groups. In the past, everyone was familiar with the other doctors in the county and had a working relationship. There was a common identity among the physicians. Problems and concerns were brought to the Medical Society and discussed. Agreement and decisions may not have always been in the best interest of the individual or the community, but there was a consensus reached and an opportunity to express opinions. The primary conduit for individuals to express their concerns at present are the multispecialty group or hospital staff. The Medical Society has less importance to the individual. Dr. Ralph Carter's view of the role of the local medical society in determining the needs of the community, the publication of a fee schedule by the society, and the requirement of society membership for practice in Brown County are in the past.

Twenty five years ago, Dr. John Dettmann acknowledged the changes taking place in medicine and his confidence in the art and practice of medicine. Fortunately, physicians continue to be motivated by the same principles that brought the frontier doctors to this area. Relieving pain and suffering, treating the sick and dying, and encouraging health are enduring endeavors of every physician. It is more difficult in today's medical community. The role of the doctor in preserving a close doctor-patient relationship with full participation by the informed patient and a sincere attempt to emphasize prevention has not changed. What has changed are the economic and business practices of medicine. Technology has driven many of the changes. It would be difficult for the Beaumonts, Minahans and Bellins of the past to adjust to today's medical practice. The physician of today has to appreciate the changes to understand his/her role in the practice of medicine in Brown County.

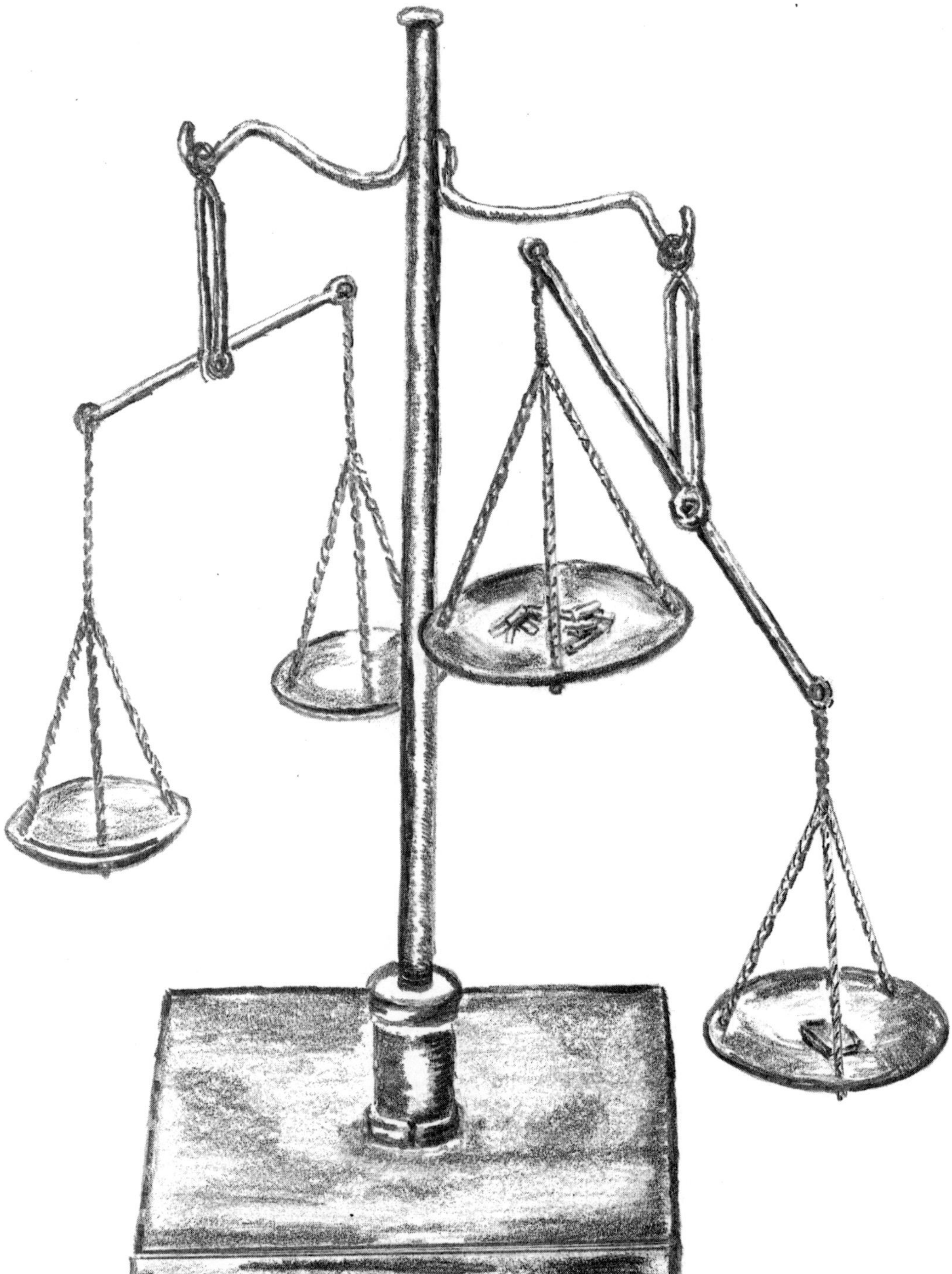

Double arm apothecary scale c. 1800

Index

Index

Index

Index

Index

Index

Index

Index

Index

Index

Index